Sherry Sweeney, OTR/L

Occupational Therapy Assessment as the Keystone to Treatment Planning

The *Occupational Therapy in Health Care* series, Florence S. Cromwell, Editor

- *The Changing Roles of Occupational Therapists in the 1980s*
- *Occupational Therapy Assessment as the Keystone to Treatment Planning*
- *Occupational Therapy and the Patient with Pain*
- *Computers, New Tools of Treatment and Practice*
- *Equipment, Bridge to Functional Independence*
- *After Treatment, What*
- *Private Practice, The Growing Model for OT Services*
- *Treatment of the Adolescent with Behavioral Problems*

Occupational Therapy Assessment as the Keystone to Treatment Planning

Florence S. Cromwell
Editor

The Haworth Press
New York

Occupational Therapy Assessment as the Keystone to Treatment Planning has also been published as *Occupational Therapy in Health Care,* Volume 1, Number 2, Summer 1984.

The Haworth Press, Inc., 28 East 22 Street, New York NY 10010

Library of Congress Cataloging in Publication Data
Main entry under title:

Occupational therapy assessment as the keystone to treatment planning.

Includes bibliographical references.
1. Occupational therapy—Evaluation—Addresses, essays, lectures. I. Cromwell, Florence S. [DNLM: 1. Occupational therapy. 2. Patient care planning—Methods.
WB 555 A846
RM735.36.028 1984 615.8'515 84-697
ISBN 0-86656-305-9

Occupational Therapy Assessment as the Keystone to Treatment Planning

Occupational Therapy in Health Care
Volume 1, Number 2

CONTENTS

JANET C. STONE, BA, OTR, *Former Department Head, Occupational Therapy, Rancho Los Amigos Hospital, Downey, California, and Initiating Editor, AOTA Bulletin on Practice, Huntington Beach, CA*

CARL SUNDSTROM, MA, OTR, LTC, AMSC, *Occupational Therapy Staff Officer, Health Services Command, Fort Sam Houston, TX*

MARY GRACE WASHBURN, MHA, OTR, FAOTA, *Marketing Director, Health Care Design Services, Kirkham, Michael and Associates, Architects, Engineers and Planners, Denver, Colorado*

CARLOTTA WELLES, MA, OTR, FAOTA, *Consultant, Professional Liability, and Former Chairman, Occupational Therapy Department, Los Angeles City College, Los Angeles, CA*

Occupational Therapy Assessment as the Keystone to Treatment Planning

FROM THE EDITOR'S DESK

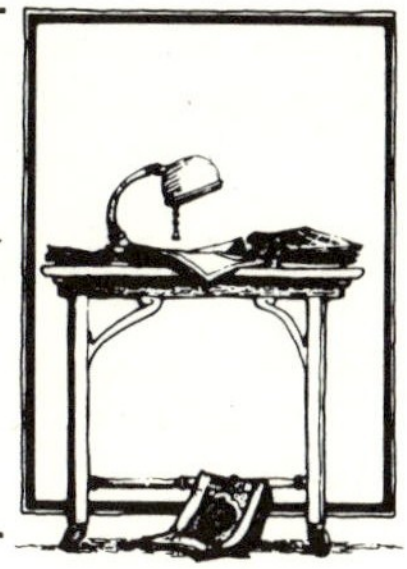

I find it difficult to be thinking in terms of a *Summer* issue of OTHC, and the second in Volume 1 at that, when we have not yet been seen by you, our potential readers. In a sense we must operate on hunches and in a reader vacuum in the start-up stages of a new journal. But by the time you see this issue you will have begun to taste the flavor of our offerings and have some reactions to them. Therefore now we solicit your comments and suggestions.

Already, in accordance with earlier promises, we are considering the addition of several vehicles for reader reaction and exchange, albeit difficult to do that in a timely fashion given the lead time for each issue. In our Fall issue we shall have a reader/reactor present his thoughts generated from a sneak preview of the papers in that issue. He will draw some inferences about the state of the profession's practice in the theme area, the treatment of pain, as well as what he may see as indications for research, new directions, education and such as reflected in those papers.

Second we hope by then to have instituted a feature that we shall call "Practice Watch" in which persons by invitation will present essays that are overviews or special perspectives or which present concerns regarding occupational therapy and the directions the field is headed. These columns will appear irregularly and usually will be unrelated in content to the theme of the issue. An extra, if you will.

This issue addresses a topic that is one of the linchpins of our practice, the what, why, how and when of the patient evaluation process. Nothing we do is more critical in determining the focus and quality of our treatment efforts than when we make the decision of what and how to evaluate patient function as the basis for all subsequent treatment activity. All clinical knowledge is for naught if we have not decided carefully what our approaches to planning shall be and have zeroed in on those aspects of function and dysfunction that will point the way to selection and use of treatment strategies. On the other hand, evaluation or assessment by itself is an exercise in futility. It does little good to probe and examine if we do not know what we are looking for and in what context we shall use the data we find.

Occupational therapists have gained significant sophistication in viewing patients' performance in life activities in order to pinpoint assets and liabilities which then become the resources and signals for our choice of treatment activities. In this issue we hope we have first helped you to look broadly at the process of evaluation as the keystone of treatment planning. Hurff helps us to do that. Then we have provided overviews of current assessment activity and philosophies in two major segments of practice, physical disabilities and mental health. The authors, each a former chair of the respective AOTA Special Interest Sections, are in a good position to provide data on both practice habits and what is perceived as the mind-set of today's practitioners on the subject of assessment.

These broad looks are followed by descriptions of a selection of specific pieces of evaluation practice or of specific instruments now in use among occupational therapists. Whether the patient has arthritis or hemiplegia, epilepsy or mental retardation, is energy deficient or simply trying to make his way, with disability, in the mainstream of study or work activities, occupational therapists have particular sensitivities to his needs. And they use assessment in the context of that philosophy to bring focus to a treatment program that will address his problems.

Our authors share their models with you in the hope that you may find them useful. They doubtless welcome your reactions and inquiry as well as your experiences similar to their own. By your sharing, another objective of our journal will be achieved—the building of a network of persons with common interests in the practice of occupational therapy.

Florence S. Cromwell
Editor

Visualization: A Decision-Making Tool for Assessment and Treatment Planning

Janith McCready Hurff, MA, OTR

ABSTRACT. This paper presents the notion that visualization can be a useful strategy for decision-making in occupational therapy practice. Model building as a way of organizing and relating the ingredients to treatment decisions is presented in a variety of forms and applied to assessment and treatment situations.

INTRODUCTION

The subtle or obvious problems patients present in the physical and/or psychological domains direct the occupational therapist's energies into the evaluation process. Gillette, in describing this activity as a 'spiral building process' indicates that treatment objectives are defined and incorporated into a treatment plan, each treatment session is reviewed for effectiveness, and then revision or modification of treatment procedures occurs as needed. However, "It is the system of evaluation which is built into the treatment process that ultimately determines the effectiveness of treatment".[1]

Medical records, observations, interviews and checklists, history taking, informal and formal assessments provide relevant information from which treatment objectives and effective clinical techniques or procedures are formulated. The evaluation or assessment process is one part of professional decision-making.

Janith McCready Hurff was Assistant Director of Training in Occupational Therapy at the University Affiliated Program, Children's Hospital of Los Angeles, Los Angeles, California, 1971-1983.

The preliminary stage of the assessment process involves manipulation of ideas, reflective thinking, cognitive comparing of potential options, and selection of a course of action. Mental imagery, or visualizing of the assessment and treatment process could be helpful to some clinicians both early and later in the treatment scheme. Visualization can be a tool to clarify which assessments to select, which frames of reference to apply to the clinical situation, which treatment strategies to employ, and finally when and how to reassess in each of these parts of the treatment process.

VISUALIZATION AS A WAY OF THINKING

The differences between visualization and verbalization of thought processes often go unrecognized. These distinctive approaches to thinking stem from different sensory worlds. Visualizers range from those individuals who possess well developed powers of imagery and who often approach problems spatially to those who have weak imagery skills and rarely use them. The visualizers who are strong problem solvers tend to produce images rich in detail, texture, containing movement, sounds, smells, and other sensory attributes. The less developed visualizers approach problems in linear, step-by-step fashion. On the other hand, verbalizers or vocalizers have an intellectual style which combines words, concepts, generalities and other abstractions to express ideas. This mode of imagery involves talking to one's self before presenting ideas rather than creating and structuring mental pictures as tools for thinking.

Very young children think predominantly in mental images which give way over time to words and abstract concepts. Sommer[2] reminds his readers that the elderly recall memories and childhood scenes with such clarity that one questions whether humans, as they age, revert back to modes of thinking that once served as their principal thinking processes. One's habits of visual or verbal imagery actually are more related to interests, occupations and cognitive style. Persons in architecture, art and engineering exercise visualization and spatial thinking while those fields which require analysis, reflection and abstraction seem to attract the verbal image thinker.[3]

A review of *The American Journal of Occupational Therapy* during the past two decades reveals the emergence of a blending of visual and verbal thinkers among authors. This is seen in the increased presentation of models throughout the articles. The building of models, or thinking visually, appears as an increasingly popular tool for occupational therapists in both theory development and in approaches to treatment.

THE MODEL: AN IMAGERY/VISUALIZATION TOOL

A model is a way of visualizing concepts and ideas and represents the parts, characteristics and relationships of a situation, condition or phenomenon.[4] It is an organizing technique designed to assist in categorizing ideas and structuring approaches to thinking about complex problems. Some models are built horizontally or vertically as in a flow chart or diagram configuration. However, the ecological holistic approach to the complexities of human behavior, such as that used by many occupational therapists, is best served by an open general systems model. That kind of model directs attention to the interactions that occur within and between component parts of the whole. The systems way of thinking can be incorporated into many forms of models. Change or progress in such models is represented through the concept of hierarchy in which higher components or subsystems are dependent upon the states of lower level subsystems.[4]

This article presents examples of ways occupational therapists can visualize ideas in order to solve treatment problems. Various conceptual models used by occupational therapists will be described as they may be applied to clinical situations and/or for conducting assessments with patients in different stages of the life cycle. Finally, suggestions will be shared about designing models for specific use in assessment and treatment planning. The process or product of model building will be illustrated by models selected from current occupational therapy literature. Because such mental representations can be valuable ways to picture or conceptualize a problem situation, their use in this presentation is intended to stimulate the reader to generate his own creative and original picture making for the identification of obstacles or objectives, to apply his store of information as it relates to the clinical problems at hand, to speculate cause-effect outcomes, and to acknowledge interactions or interrelationships of importance. These conceptual tools or ways of thinking can be designed using many forms: a spiral, circle, with lines or dynamically.

TYPES OF MODELS

Spiral Imagery

Visualization of human development and the identification of areas needing occupational therapy intervention may be viewed in many configurations. However, a spiral model is often used to illustrate the principles of growth and development. In it the dynamic process of human development is shown, i.e., that (a) development is orderly, predictable and sequential, (b) individuals differ in when changes occur though still within a normal continuum of development, (c) expectations imposed by others affect growth and development, (d) individual areas of development may show uneven gains *within* various stages of maturation, and (e) development fluctuates between equilibrium and disequilibrium over time.[5]

Ames developed a spiral model progressing upward in increasingly larger circles representing child development from 18 months to 6 years. The spiral configuration enabled her to present in the levels of the spiral the time periods of 18 months, 2½, 3½, 4½, 5½ to 6 years as times of disequilibrium. The years of 2, 3, 4 and 5, on the other hand, are illustrated as plateaus and of equilibrium.[6] Others have used a spiraling continuum model to show the development of spatiotemporal adaptation. Their visualization helps the viewer to see the progression of development starting when sensory input is assimilated, which leads to motor output and the process of accommodation, then sensory feedback which affects how one associates/differentiates, and ends in adaptation when the person is automatically able to change appropriately to spatial demands.[5] In using a spiral representation of developmental change the treatment planner is able to account for the patient's growth spurts as well as for those sometimes worrisome plateaus when time is needed to assimilate and adapt to new experiences and learning.

Circular Visualization

Problem solving may also be facilitated by using circular imagery. A biopsychosocial model for occupational therapy practice was introduced by Mosey as an alternative to the use of a medical or health model.[7] Another representation of occupational therapy practice in circular form was presented by the Task Force on Target Populations.[8] Figure 1 presents this model.

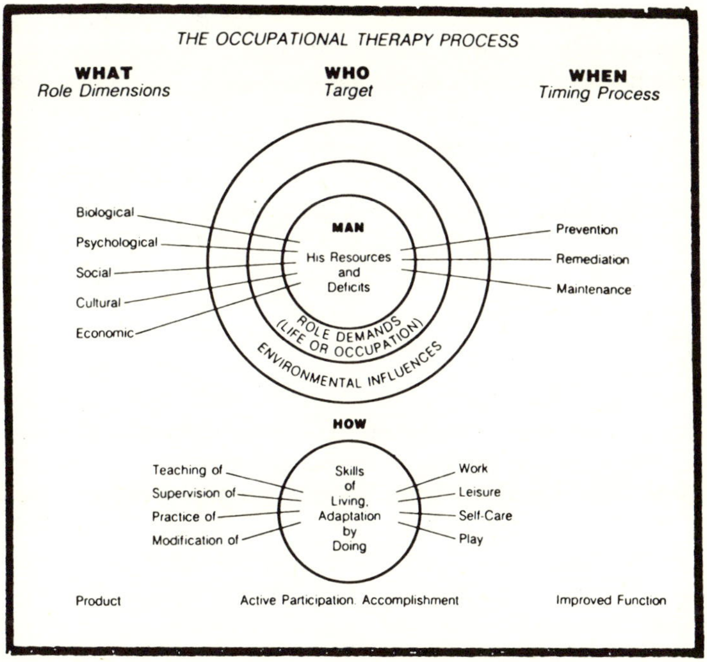

FIGURE 1. Reprinted with permission of American Occupational Therapy Association, Inc., copyright 1974, Am J Occ Ther, Vol 28 No 3, March 1974, p 161.

Howe and Briggs designed a circular conceptual model which they present as an ecological systems model. By visualizing the individual as an open system, they felt the examiner could direct attention to the individual, to his environment and to the dynamic processes of interaction between them. The ecological systems model is pictured in a series of nested layers indicating the person's immediate setting, social networks and institutions, and ideological system (social and cultural values). Intervention with the patient is then guided by what one notes in assessing the interactions among these layers in which life tasks, roles and life skills are major considerations. In this frame of reference one's attention is directed both to factors contributing to dysfunction and the constraints on health as well as to the factors present which support healthy functioning.[9]

Still in the circular form Clark proposed a model for occupational therapy practice which blends four theoretical approaches: adaptive performance (Fidler and Mosey), biodevelopmental (Ayres, Willbarger and others), facilitating growth and development (Llorens) and occupational behavior (Reilly). The model is generated from a view of the profession, a view of man as an adaptive being and a view of health as the focus for intervention.[10] The domains of self maintenance, play and work are incorporated into overlapping, related circles to create an organizing visualization of occupational therapy practice. Figure 2 illustrates Clark's model. An important feature of circular imagery in occupational therapy is that it assists the therapist to view the patient in a more holistic manner. This attention can result in more thorough, comprehensive treatment planning and intervention.

Linear Imagery

Linear models are visualizations most commonly seen as flow charts, diagrams, matrices and organizational charts. As such they are useful as organizers in planning and management, e.g., time

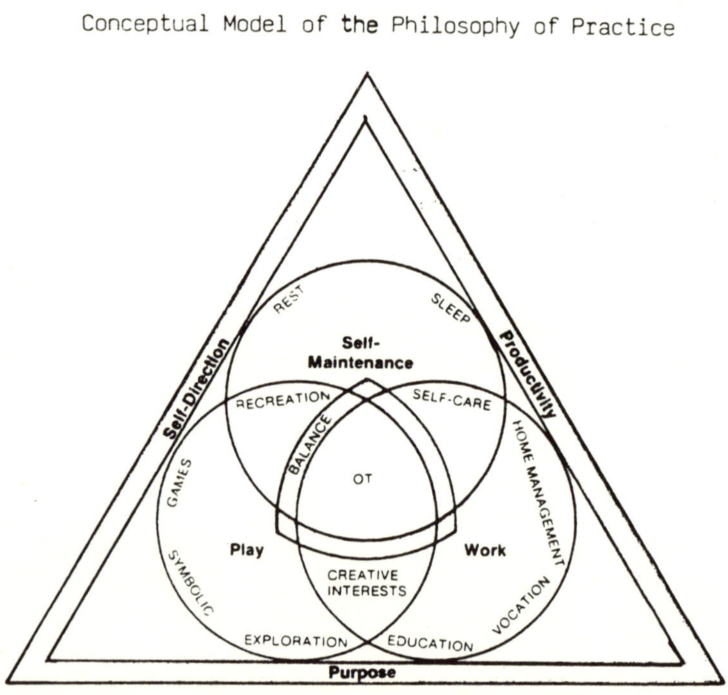

FIGURE 2. Reprinted with permission of The American Occupational Therapy Association, Inc., copyright 1979, Am J Occ Ther, Vol 33 No 9, September 1979, p 518.

planning and production control. In occupational therapy many evaluations of play behavior are available in matrix (chart or box) form to guide clinical observation.[11] For use in mental health treatment Allen introduced a chart with a hierarchy of cognitive levels and task analyses for cognitive disability applicable in understanding varied levels of mental illness.[12] Allen's model promises to be an extremely useful tool for viewing complex clinical puzzles.

Dynamic Representations

An open system model from general systems theory enables the clinician to visualize overall human functioning. In it the dynamics of the interrelationships and interactions between its parts and from outside the system (the environment) are represented. The constructs of input, throughput, output and feedback comprise the framework of an open system and can readily be built for clinical situations in occupational therapy from what one knows or needs to know or must assess about a patient and his current problem. *Input* represents the internal and external information received into the system for operation, such as the patient's functional limitations, intellectual and emotional status and personal values. *Throughput* is the processing of the input such as one's making adjustments in doing daily activities to fit his own living situation. *Output* is the product or outcome of performance. The *feedback* mechanisms serve to monitor behavior of the system and its parts and results in cueing of status quo or for change. Figure 3 illustrates this model.

The notion of hierarchy as used in general systems theory and modeling is also an organizing and analyzing tool for occupational therapists to use in clinical practice since the rules of hierarchy can account for changes that occur in a system (in a patient's behavior, for example). Attention must be addressed to the maintenance of lower levels of function which are the underpinnings of higher levels of behavior. When damage or disruption occurs at lower levels of function higher levels are necessarily affected.[13] Play behavior has often been described in hierarchical stages. Each stage is a progression from a lower to a higher level of curiosity or excitement and refinement.[11] Figure 4 exemplifies these interrelationships. To elaborate, exploratory play is free play engaged in for pleasure as the child learns rules about self, the environment, objects and people. In competency behavior one develops skills to deal with and to trust the environment and these evolve into self concepts

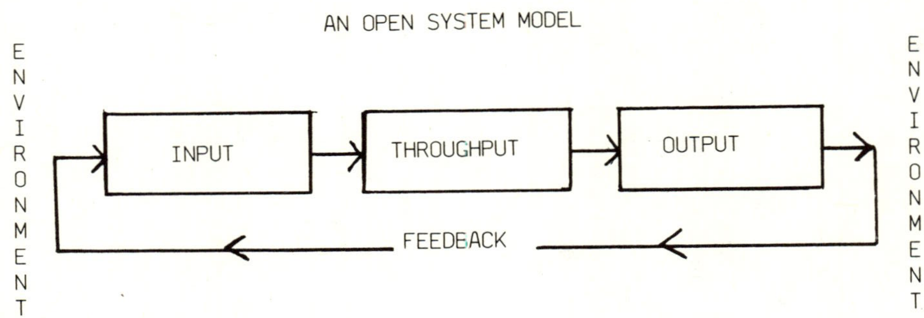
AN OPEN SYSTEM MODEL
ENVIRONMENT
INPUT
THROUGHPUT
OUTPUT
ENVIRONMENT
FEEDBACK

FIGURE 3.

Hierarchy of Play Development

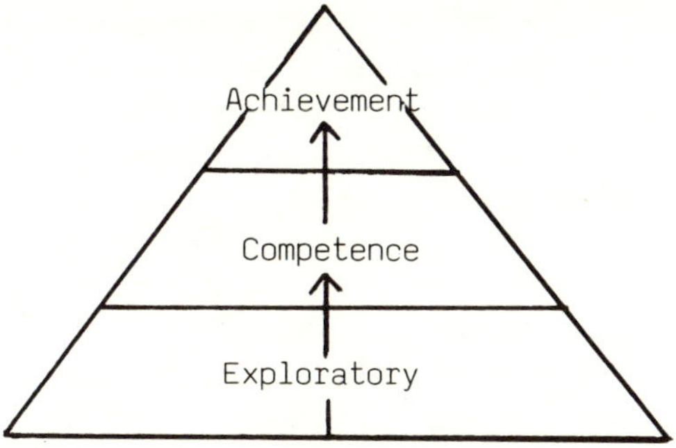

FIGURE 4.

and self-confidence. Achievement behavior emphasizes performance, mastery over the environment through risk taking, development of courage and a sense of competition. Each of the higher stages is dependent upon having acquired the behaviors in the stage(s) preceding it. Thus visualizations using hierarchical stages can illustrate the process by which primitive, simpler behaviors are transformed to newer and more complex behaviors. The process of change or the relationships of one level to the next which transforms behavior can be shown as quantitative change (simple to complex, small to large) or qualitative change (lower to higher, immature to refined). A comprehensive hierarchical model of human occupation has evolved from those using the occupational behavior frame of reference in treatment. This model is another example of an open system visualization designed to assist in directing occupational therapy assessment and intervention.[14]

In summary, the foundation of skills needed for competent functioning can be organized and conceptualized through models with an hierarchical format. Such mental representations of thinking direct the therapist's attention to areas of function appropriate for assessment and remediation. They may in fact point out specific areas needing occupational therapy intervention that might not otherwise be considered. Thus it can be seen that the therapist using an hierarchical model might optimize the use of both clinical and home environments by specifying the task demands necessary to nurture desired behavioral outcomes.

APPROACHES TO ASSESSMENT

Many approaches to treatment are used by occupational therapists. Three approaches frequently mentioned are developmental, habilitation/rehabilitation and occupational behavior.[5] The organizing principles which guide these and other approaches to treatment are called frames of reference.

A frame of reference in occupational therapy specifies the perimeters of intervention strategies. The targets of practice selected dictate the types of activities used in treatment. A knowledge base, treatment concepts and a basic philosophy about occupational therapy dictate which frame(s) of reference one uses. Choice of a particular frame of reference is influenced by the clinical puzzles posed by the patient, the philosophy of the agency in which treatment occurs, and the bias/expertise of the therapist.[5]

For example, a developmental approach may be a neurodevelopmental perspective as used by Bobath, a neurophysiological perspective characterized by Rood techniques, an adaptive perspective as developed by Mosey, the proprioceptive neuromuscular facilitation (PNF) perspective of Kabat, Knott and Voss, a neuromuscular reflex perspective such as Fay-Doman-Delacato propose, a sensory integration perspective developed by Ayres or a neurobehavioral perspective as described by Neufred and Williamson.[5] Many frames of reference overlap and therapists can freely draw from several so long as they adhere to the organizing principles of each.

On the other hand, the habilitation/rehabilitation approach to treatment directs efforts towards restoration of ability to function in daily roles. This approach focuses strongly on development of particular skills of daily living. In the previous approaches normal movement patterns, increased sensory integration, improved developmental skills and adaptation to environment are the goals. Common among the techniques used by therapists using these frames of reference are manipulation of sensory input to control or enhance motor output, the focus on purposeful patterns of movement as organizers for the central nervous system, application of developmental principles in selecting activities, concern for reflex integration, and utilization of neurological feedback concepts. A model reflecting parts of this approach is seen in Figure 5.

The occupational behavior frame of reference is concerned with the problems of adaptation which confront a dysfunctional person. Adaptation is a complex process requiring that one possess the com-

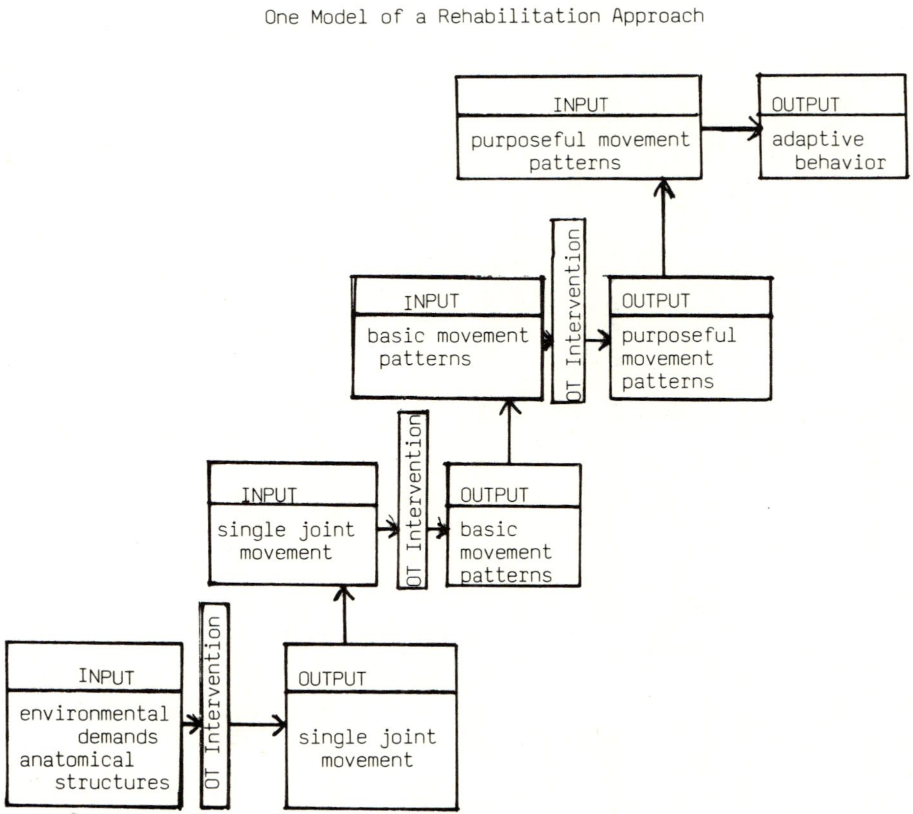

FIGURE 5. Model based upon material from the Occupational Therapy Department, University of Southern California. Author unknown.

petency behaviors that will match the demands of daily living. Instead of focusing on symptom reduction, therapists using this frame of reference emphasize daily living activities and balanced use of time in work, play, rest and sleep. Acquisition of functional skills and habits, motivation towards competency, and performance of occupational roles (preschooler, student, housewife, husband, father, worker, retiree) are critical concerns addressed over a continuum from childhood to old age.[5] An illustration of such a model is presented in Figure 6.[15]

As was noted, several frames of reference can be used simultaneously or sequentially in clinical practice. Williamson describes the example of therapy for a developmentally disabled child in which the clinician may draw upon the theories of neurodevelopment, Piaget, learning or other theoretical bodies of knowledge of treatment to plan the treatment.[16] Only with a philosophical perspective guiding the focus of clinical attention can the therapist begin the mental manipulation of clinical data to find potential solutions to patient problems be they neurodevelopmental, neurophysiological, sensory integrative or of role dysfunction and/or psychiatric or behavioral aberrations.

WHY MODELS

The saying, 'a picture is worth a thousand words' applies quite appropriately to situations within occupational therapy practice. Because a model guides and organizes one's thinking and provides a way to understand the complexities in a simpler way, it can be a supportive technique for the new clinician or for the therapist who enters a clinical setting outside his own specialization. For example, some of the models selected for this writing are general models to guide program development (Figures 2, 5, 6, 7) and can be applied to varied clinical settings and to patient populations of various ages and disabilities. Or models can be designed to address specific areas of intervention (Figures 5, 7, 8) and suggest specific assessment and treatment needs and strategies. Occupational therapists serving as academic educators and clinical instructors frequently find the use of models a valuable teaching strategy particularly when defining and illustrating the occupational therapy process (e.g., Figures 1, 2).

An Occupational Behavior Model

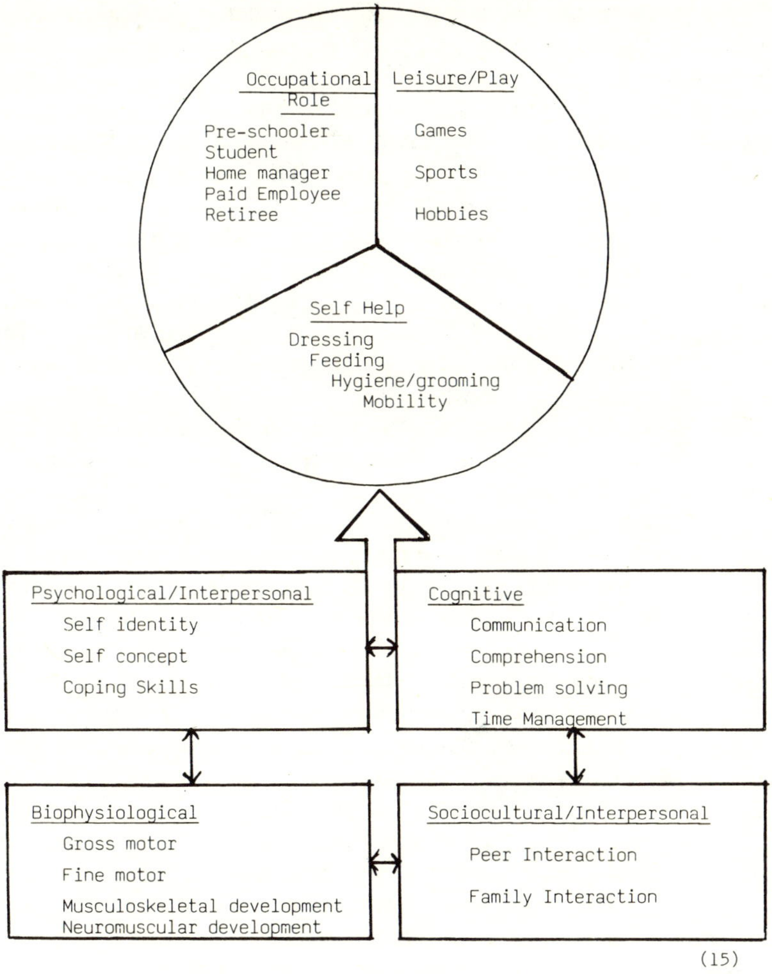

FIGURE 6.

HOW TO CONSTRUCT MODELS

How does the clinician choose what goes into the boxes or circles when he decides to formulate an idea into a model? What style best represents the clinical problem at hand? How are relationships between components of the model to be represented? How can the process of change be described? The starting point is the identification of the phenomena, from which the designer will work BACKWARDS. Think, for example, that the problem is the occupational therapy process with the goal of adaptation and of all the components which might contribute to that goal. Since the model is a thinking tool it must visually represent relationships among its parts as well as the dynamics within the whole. Such a framework can be pictured in any of the previously discussed formats or even in a combination of all. Thus the conceptualizer must be a designer who identifies components that are relevant to the understanding or description of the phenomena, as of the example cited. These constructs can then be boxed, framed, circled, stacked or encased in any form for incorporation and integration into the model framework. They may stand alone or be categorized.

But as the designer/thinker, the model builder arranges parts to show how he perceives the phenomena at hand. The categories representing the various contributing factors are then analyzed and broken down into smaller subdivisions. This is done by thinking backwards from complex to simple, large to small, higher level to lower level functioning, fine to gross behaviors or refined to immature actions. Change is represented by hierarchical configurations. Lower functioning must precede higher functions. The loss or disruption of the lower hierarchy will prevent or distort the functioning of the higher level of performance. The lower levels, or subroutines, are interactive or dynamic in the sense that each affects the other over time. The model can be constructed so that it can identify gaps, deficits, weaknesses or strengths within the framework.

In designing a model for human functioning one must provide for the influences of environment, how they interact with and within the person and what behaviors result and return to the environment. This kind of dynamic process must be accommodated by an open system in which feedback provides the mechanism and stimulus for modification and change.

AN EXAMPLE OF DESIGNING A MODEL

The Model of Middle Childhood (Figure 7)[17] illustrates the development and functioning characteristics of this life stage. A visualization such as this of this life stage could serve as an effective road

MODEL OF MIDDLE CHILDHOOD

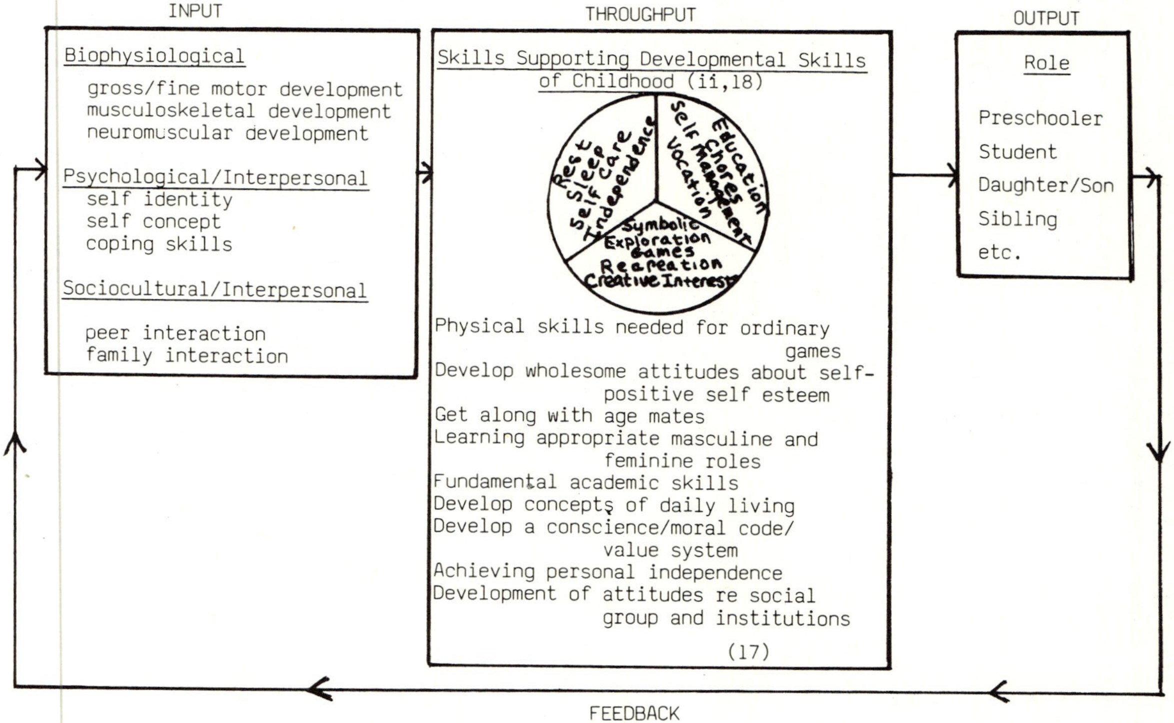

FIGURE 7.

map for a therapist. It could also act as a checklist of important areas to be considered during the assessment and treatment process. The model is an open systems approach such as described in Figure 3. The input section suggests the need for the therapist to assess the many factors comprising the child's biophysiological, psychological and sociocultural functioning. The throughput section represents the child's processing and acquisition of the skills required during middle childhood. The output section guides the therapist to analyze the child's function in his various roles. The feedback occurs in the child's awareness or learning that recognition for him can be gained through competence and mastery of his interactions with tools, objects and people. If the therapist finds evidence, for example, that the child has a poor self image or low self esteem in any of his roles, this directs attention to the feedback process and should lead the therapist to assess causes such as motivational factors which might include his expectancies of success or failure, his internal versus external orientation, his 'belief in skill' and his sense of 'efficacy'.[18, 19]

Working further backwards as the model suggests the therapist would pose various questions. Is school performance at age expectancy? Is there a delay or lag in self help skills or overall independence? Is the child withdrawn or lacking in the ability to interact with peers? Is he a disruptive family member? Such questions relate to role behavior and lead the investigation still further backwards to identify those developmental skills prerequisite to role acquisition. As the therapist moves backward in this manner in the analysis and assessment of dysfunction his own mental imagery then begins to move the past and present pieces of clinical evidence into focus and into perspective with the whole. Is there a gap or deficit in play skills? Has there been deprivation in decision making opportunities and activities? Is the presenting problem acute or chronic? What physical or behavioral areas require training, retraining or support? A visual framework or model can in this way also assist the therapist/evaluator to attend to specific needs such as splinting, range of motion, positioning, muscle strengthening or muscle reeducation, sensory-integrative needs or other areas of occupational therapy concern within the complexity of the total person.

The Development of Occupational Choice model (Figure 8) is one particularly applicable for use in treating patients in adolescence and adulthood. The task of occupational choice is central in adolescence and depends upon the child possessing a baseline of prerequisite skills and abilities acquired during middle childhood. Occupational choice is a decision making action occurring over a period of years and involves making choices among one's interests and abilities against the realities and demands of the work world.[20] Because being able to work and gain satisfaction from work is such a fundamental concern of occupational therapists, a model of occupational choice can be a very practical guide to therapists treating adolescents and young adult patients regardless of the setting.

Ginzberg described the process of occupational choice as occurring in three stages that can take place or be recapitulated throughout the life span: the Fantasy Period (generally ending by age 11), the Tentative Stage (during ages 11-17) and the Realistic Period (from age 17 through adulthood). Each period is characterized by the nature of the choices during that stage. The hierarchy of the occupational choice process is presented in Figure 8.

Therapists working from an occupational choice model may find the Geist Picture Interest Inventory[21] useful as an assessment of vocational interests. It is a pictorial test which quantitatively identifies interests and motivational forces behind occupational choice. Findings from this assessment can be mapped onto the occupational choice model shown to identify either delays or age appropriate functioning of the patient tested. The visualization of the occupational choice process pinpoints specific areas of function (transitional skills) which may require attention or those stages into which the individual may be moving. Findings from engaging in this kind of assessment have proven clinically useful particularly as input to interdisciplinary team evaluation conferences, for parent counseling and school consultations.

SUMMARY AND CONCLUSIONS

Visualization is a thinking process that can enhance the efficacy of assessment and problem solving in treatment planning in occupational therapy by making clear the many components that must be considered in treatment depending on the frame(s) of reference used. The process can picture and define in term of one's frame of reference the relationships of all the ingredients to treatment in order to organize the direction of both assessment and treatment strategies. Models help one to view the individual patient and his problems as an open system and direct the therapist's attention to the presence and/or absence of normal functioning or to the impacts on

THE DEVELOPMENT OF OCCUPATIONAL CHOICE

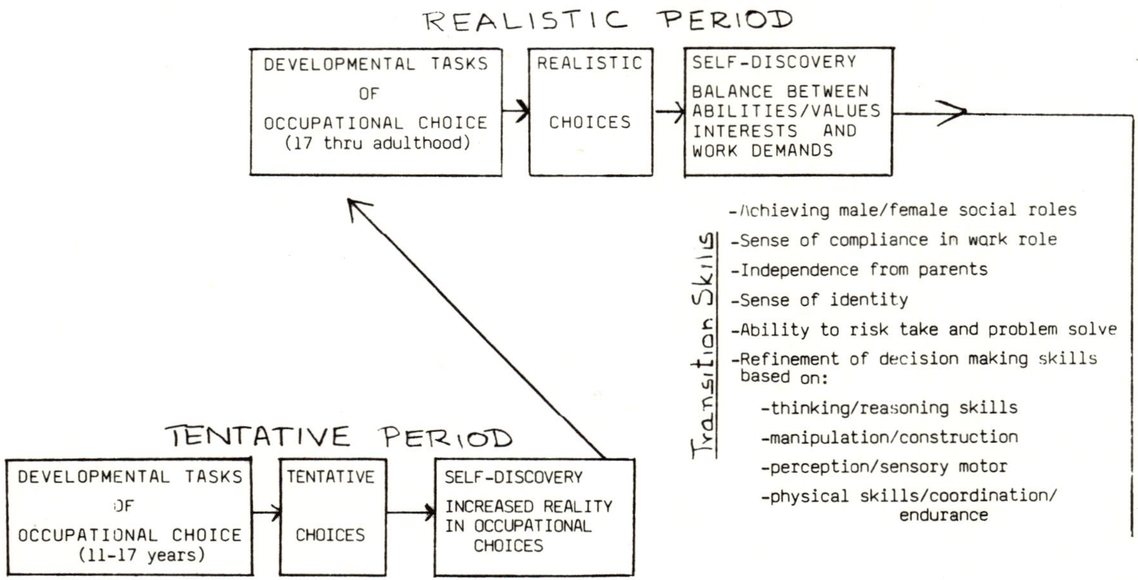

FIGURE 8.

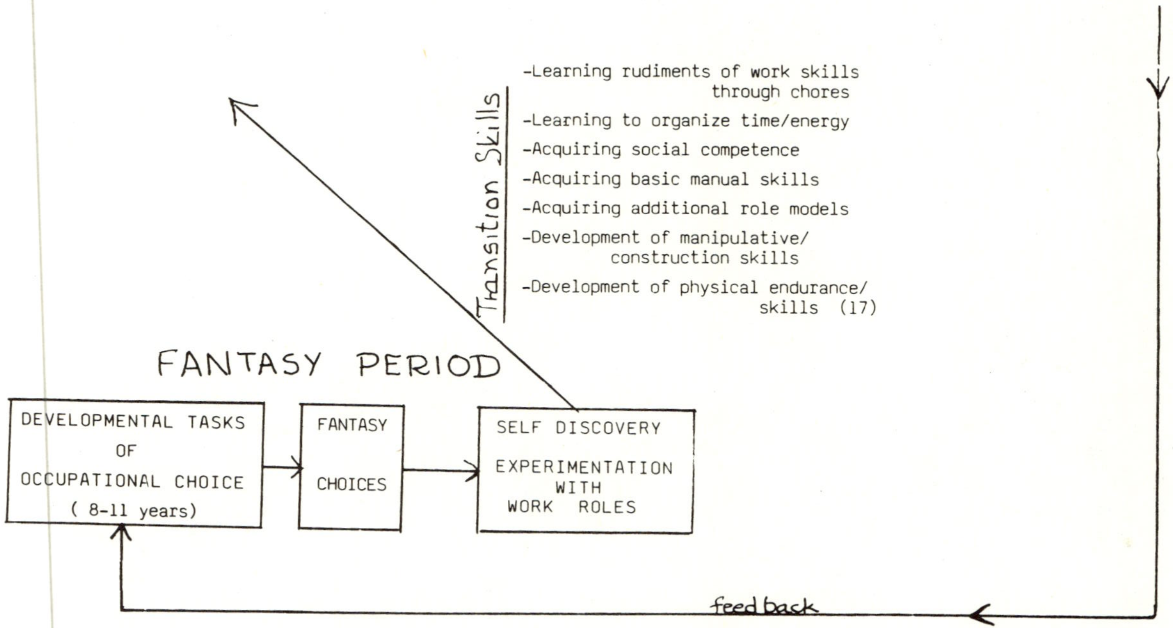

REENTRY BACK INTO OCCUPATIONAL CHOICE PROCESS AT ANY LEVEL TO EXPLORE ALTERNATIVES AND OTHER VOCATIONAL OPTIONS

FIGURE 8, continued.

function from the course of disease. One then is able to choose the appropriate assessments and justify their use as a result of having mentally manipulated (using the model as a guide) and determined the breakdowns of inputs (routines into subsystems, skills into subskills and requisites into prerequisites) necessary to pinpoint treatment goals and the routes to them. A variety of model configurations have been presented which illustrate how this can occur.

Because the occupational therapist views the patient as an integrated whole, models, being holistic, guide the therapist to identify logically the multiple areas of function that must be examined and to develop an action plan based upon the patient's strengths as well as his problems. Short and long term goals can be pictured, prioritized and incorporated into a treatment plan for implementation. Visualization is a tool which permits one to speculate cause-effect outcomes, to juggle clinical puzzles, to explore interactions or interrelationships occurring during assessment and/or treatment and to review the effectiveness of treatment. The visualizing process begins again in the spiral building fashion described by Gillette as revisions and modifications of treatment procedures occur.

Using visualization in the form of model building is an appropriate tool for occupational therapy decision making. It provides many variations and options for the therapist to use when approaching the complexities of clinical assessment and treatment planning.

BIBLIOGRAPHY

1.Gillette, N.: Occupational Therapy and Mental Health. In Willard, H.S., and Spackman, C.S. (eds.): *Occupational Therapy,* ed. 4, Philadelphia, J.B. Lippincott Co., 1971, p. 79.

2. Sommer, R.: *The Mind's Eye-Imagery in Everyday Life,* Delacorte Press, New York, 1978.

3. Bray, A.: *Directing the Movies of Your Mind,* Harper and Row, New York, 1978.

4. Boulding, K.: *The Image-Knowledge in Life and Society,* Ann Arbor Paperbacks, University of Michigan Press, 1971.

5. Hopkins, H.L., and Smith, H.D .: *Willard and Spackman's Occupational Therapy,* Fifth Edition, Philadelphia, J.B. Lippincott Co., 1978.

6. Ames, L.B.: *Child Care and Development,* Philadelphia, J.P. Lippincott Co., 1978, p. 5.

7. Mosey, A.C.: An Alternative: The Biopsychosocial Model. In *Am. J. Occup. Ther.,* Vol. 28, No. 3, March 1974, p. 137.

8. Task Force on Target Populations. In *Am. J. Occup. Ther.,* Vol. 28, No. 3, March 1974, p. 161.

9. Howe, M., and Briggs, A.: The Ecological Systems Model for Occupational Therapy. In *Am. J. Occup. Ther.,* Vol. 36, No. 5, May 1982, pp. 322-327.

10. Clark. P.: Human Development through Occupation: A Philosophy and Conceptual Model for Practice, Part 2. In *Am. J. Occup. Ther.,* vol. 33, No. 9, Sept. 1979, p. 518.

11. Reilly, M.: *Play as Exploratory Learning,* Sage Publications, Beverly Hills, 1974.

12. Allen, C.: Independence through Activities: The Practice of Occupational Therapy. In *Am. J. Occup. Ther.,* Vol. 36, No. 11, November 1982.

13. Kielhofner, G.: A Paradigm for Practice: The Hierarchical Organization of Occupational Therapy Knowledge. In *Health through Occupation,* Kielhofner, (ed.), Philadelphia, F.A. Davis, 1983, p. 85.

14. Kielhofner, G., and Burke, J.: A Model of Human Occupation, Part 1. In *Am. J. Occup. Ther.,* Vol. 34, No. 9, Sept. 1980. pp. 572-581.

15. Nuesca, A.: Presentation made at the University Affiliated Program, Childrens Hospital of Los Angeles, December 1981.

16. Williamson, G.: A Heritage of Activity: Development of Theory. In *Am. J. Occup. Ther.,* Vol. 36, No. 11, Nov. 1982.

17. Havighurst, R.: *Developmental Tasks and Education,* 2nd ed., David McKay Co., Inc., New York, 1969.

18. Hurff, J.: *Protecting the Achievement Behavior and Competency Development of the Ten Year Old Child.* Unpublished master's thesis, University of Southern California, February 1972.

19. Burke, J.: A Clinical Perspective on Motivation: Pawn versus Origin. In *Am. J. Occup. Ther.,* Vol. 31, No. 4, April 1977, pp. 254-258.

20. Ginzberg, E., Ginzberg, S.W., Axelrod, S., and Herma, J.L.: *Occupational Choice: An Approach to General Theory,* Columbia University Press, New York, 1956.

21. Geist, H.: *The Geist Picture Interest Inventory: Male or Female,* Western Psychological Services, Los Angeles, 1968.

Assessment: The Keystone of Treatment Planning

Alice M. Bowker, MA, OTR

ABSTRACT. The role of the occupational therapist in today's health care system is discussed in relation to the large numbers of patients with treatment problems and the relatively small numbers in the profession. The importance of good, efficient assessment procedures is emphasized in order to maximize the profession's helpfulness. Review of current practices among occupational therapists in carrying out the assessment function is presented along with data from a survey of therapists in physical disabilities practice. The article concludes with a plea for the increased use of standardized evaluation tools by occupational therapists to both make their efforts more effective and to build credibility for the services of the profession.

In the competitive drive within today's health care system in which providers must give fast and effective service with the best possible results, it becomes essential for occupational therapists as members of that system to identify early in the referral process which patients have sufficient potential to make occupational therapy intervention a worthwhile effort for the patient. It is equally important that occupational therapists do not see themselves as able to provide services that are 'all things to all men', but can be selective in their choices of both patients and treatment techniques. Thus they should be able to define which techniques are effective, over what periods of time and at what point efforts should be interrupted as further gains fail to appear.

Examining the yield of patients from but one disability in the United States, cerebral vascular accidents or strokes, all providers are faced with health care problems of overwhelming magnitude.

Alice M. Bowker is Assistant Professor, Occupational Therapy Department, Florida International University, Tamiami Campus, Miami, FL. She was national chairperson of the AOTA Physical Disabilities Special Interest Section from 1978-80.

There are 500,000 new patients with stroke in the U.S. each year, and at any given time the total population with stroke is approximately 2,000,000.[1] Occupational therapists in the U.S. at present number only 36,000. It behooves them therefore, in this case as members of the stroke care team, not only to develop truly effective treatment strategies for helping to restore function to the greatest possible number of these persons with stroke disability, but also to be able to pinpoint their problems that are amenable to occupational therapy. This means precise assessment initially and throughout treatment to be certain that treatment measures are effective and correctly focused. Such careful evaluation, with any patient regardless of disability, goes a long way both in benefitting patients and their families but also in utilizing most effectively the limited numbers of occupational therapists where they can be most helpful.

THE OCCUPATIONAL THERAPIST: A SPECIALIST

The occupational therapist by education is eminently qualified to observe, explain, judge human performance. Whether one's acquired specialty is in understanding hand function, neuromuscular activities, observing patients in activities of daily living or doing vocational tasks, the occupational therapist must always compare the residual functions he observes with normal function, contrast the positive aspects of behavior with the negative in order to arrive at an estimate of patient potential for functional improvement. These decisions are made against the characteristics of the injury or disease process the patient demonstrates.

The way occupational therapists learn to think makes them well suited to this job, but the therapist must achieve credibility by accumulating proof that past judgements and actions have been effective in helping patients. Without proof treatment decisions are limited to simple obvious judgements that might be made by an astute observer. To achieve credibility the occupational therapist needs to show that his treatment decisions are based on sound data used appropriately.

METHODS OF ASSESSMENT

Various tools and techniques are used by occupational therapists in assessing patient function (Figure 1). Many therapists may not use standardized evaluations, but rely on history taking, interviews,

Observation

Anecdotal Records

Cummulative Records

Rating Scales

Self Report Forms

Sociometric Devices

Psychological Tests

Standardized Tests and Inventories

Interviews

History Taking

Figure 1. Tools and Techniques Used in Assessment by Occupational Therapists AOTA, PDSIS Survey 1979

checklists. Few occupational therapists are initially well trained in using standardized tests. Historically therapists have worked on a one-to-one basis with patients and rarely until recently used systematic evaluation to collect data for analysis to determine the effectiveness of their efforts.[2] The occupational therapist of today in treatment planning appears to use one of two kinds of clinical judgements, that of clinical intuition or that based on a definite treatment model or philosophy in which decision making is based on relevant data from tests to ascertain patient needs and treatment goals. The latter method with organized observations provides primary data for treatment planning, may pinpoint critical information about the disease process that affects both current and future functioning of the patient. This then both helps the patient to anticipate his needs and forms the basis for the therapist's clinical decision making.

There is much to be said for the more informal and qualitative kinds of evaluation in behavioral fields such as occupational therapy. They can produce in-depth data not possible to obtain with more structured instruments. These types of evaluation also offer the unique quality of being widely applicable and allow the therapist to choose and adapt them to the particular situation of each patient. They are often unfortunately also time-consuming and therefore become extremely costly to patients. Therefore therapists must be sensitive to choosing assessment strategies that are *both* treatment and cost effective.

Today's therapist must enter the evaluation process well prepared, knowing beforehand what questions to ask and how to get the best answers regardless of the instruments being used. Therapists are frequently faced with patients with multiple problems. An example would be the person with brain lesion resulting in multifaceted neurological defects along with other factors contributing to his disability such as obesity, heart disease and old age. Therapists faced with this patient showing many symptoms and disabilities such as aphasias, memory deficits, decreased ability to concentrate as well as physical limitations requires an evaluation that is systematic, heirarchical and based on clear understandings and expectations of the patient's potentials. Also as evaluator the occupational therapist must be prepared to incorporate the knowledge of many body systems as they affect function and choose tests which pinpoint both assets and deficits. Information vital to decision making needs to be efficiently procured to prevent needless frustration on the patient's part.

TESTS WITH QUANTIFIABLE YIELDS

Many occupational therapy departments are now developing and using assessment batteries for various patient groups to identify both functional levels and needs. Standardized tests which provide acknowledged measures of comparison by quantitative and/or qualitative data are increasingly evident in these batteries. Obviously the major purpose of testing, however done, is to evaluate patients' skills and abilities, as well as deficits, as a basis for treatment planning. Testing also should provide some measure of prediction so that treatment strategies can be selected and used judiciously.

While many therapists still do not use standardized evaluation procedures, and few tests within occupational therapy are available and widely used, some new assessments are beginning to appear. Further there is evidence that more therapists seek to organize and quantify their evaluations.[3] The development of tests and other methods of assessment that accurately quantify and predict functional levels of given patient groups is a Herculean task. However, through such efforts therapists may pool resources and plan programs that will lead to more effective, accepted and recognized treatment. Indeed to establish the uniqueness of occupational therapy expertise which is not readily provided by any other health care professionals, therapists must engage in accumulating and using reliable data about patient function, before and during treatment. In addition they must back up that data with valid information about outcomes that can be replicated in occupational therapy clinics around the country. In order to accomplish this urgent objective occupational therapists must forthwith acquire knowledge about testing, about selecting tests and using data acquired for diagnostic purposes to apply within the acknowledged frames of reference for treatment used within the profession.

OCCUPATIONAL THERAPY TESTING: CURRENT PRACTICE

In 1979 the American Occupational Therapy Association Specialty Sections conducted surveys among practicing occupational therapists asking, among other things, what types of evaluation tools they used in practice. Narrative indices of the tests reported in the surveys have been developed by both the Physical Disabilities and Mental Health Sections. The Physical Disabilities Index reflects 490 responses from therapists country-wide. As reported in a recent AOTA publication[3] standardized tests used by therapists treating patients with physical disabilities include seven major categories of tests. They are achievement, development, intelligence, manual dexterity, motor function, sensori-motor function and vocational interests/skills (Figure 2). The names of specific tests reported as currently used are in the areas itemized in Figure 3. By far the greatest number of tests reported are of manual dexterity and sensori-motor function.

The survey seems to show a growing trend, however, for therapists to document clinical findings through use of some structured instruments that are valid and reliable. Evaluation can point the way to more discriminating application of treatment strategies so this broader test use is encouraging for the profession. It is of course practical for therapists in their clinics and practice to develop techniques of assessment that match their patients' needs and their own frames of reference for treatment. It is also usual that they will use tests that are readily available. If valid, reliable and pertinent instruments are available for collecting desired information, better judgements in treatment will be made from using them. However, instruments should not be used indiscriminately just because they are available. If one wants usable answers to patient problems one must know which questions to ask. This then is where therapist judgement is critically tested and often results in developing one's own protocols for assessment.[4]

SUMMARY

The use of some standardized tests along with unstandardized instruments is a scheme that has been followed by occupational therapists for many years. Lacking many tests that are specific to

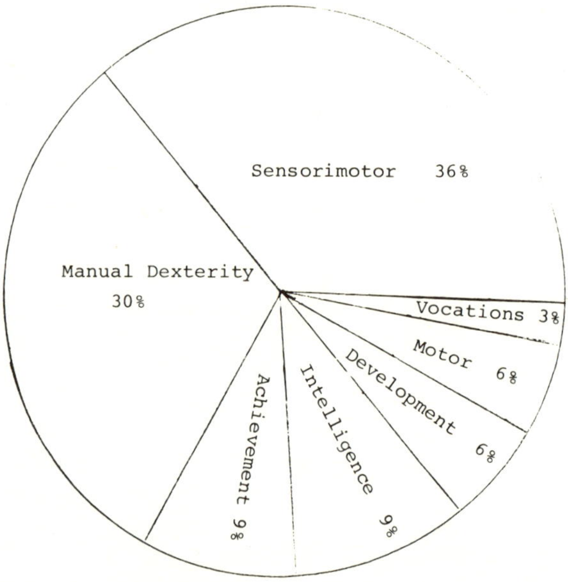

Figure 2

Categories of standardized tests used by 490 occupational therapists in physical disability clinical practice AOTA, PDSIS Survey, 1979

Achievement

Adult Basic Learning Examination
General Aptitude Test Battery
Wide Range Achievement Test

Development

Bayley Scales of Infant Development
Denver Developmental Screening Test

Intelligence

Knox Cube Test
Peabody Picture Vocabulary Test
Wechsler Adult Intelligence Scale

Manual Dexterity

Crawford Small Parts Dexterity Test
Hand Tool Dexterity Test, Bennet
Jebson-Taylor Hand Function Test
MacQuarrie Test of Mechanical Ability
Minnesota Rate of Manipulation Test
O'Connor Tweezer Dexterity Test
Pennsylvania Bi-Manual Worksample
Physical Capacities Evaluation of Hand Skill
Purdue Pegboard
Stromberg Dexterity Test

Motor

Bruininks-Oseretsky Test of Motor Proficiency
Scott Test of Motor Impairment

Sensorimotor

Beery/Buktenia Developmental Test of Visual Motor Integration
Benton Test of Visual Organization
Elizur Test of Psycho-Organicity
Frostig Developmental Test of Visual Perception
Hooper Visual Organization Test
Motor-Free Visual Perceptual Test
Raven Progressive Matrices
Sherman Mental Impairment Test
Slossen Drawing Coordination Test
Southern California Sensory Integration Tests
Symbol Digit Modalities Test
Winter Haven Visual Retention Test

Vocations

California Occupational Preference Survey

Figure 3 Standardized tests used by 490 occupational therapists in physical disability clinical practice
AOTA,PDSIS Survey, 1979

occupational therapy, therapists have sought and used tests from many other disciplines. Only now is the profession formalizing some of its own. Professionals in schools and corporations have long found that better decision making results from the use of good tests.[2] An occupational therapist equipped with test batteries relevant to both patient population and setting as well as to his treatment philosophy is better able to provide comprehensive, pertinent and predictive evaluation so necessary for treatment planning.

Assessment is the keystone to treatment planning. It is the foundation for goal setting, for selection of treatment strategies, for continually monitoring patient reaction and progress in treatment. The ability to select correct tools, to use them appropriately, and apply the data gained meaningfully in addressing patient needs and goals is after all the 'bottom line' in providing effective treatment.

REFERENCES

1. McCollough, NC: *Incidence and Functional Prognosis of the Hemiplegia,* Instructional Course Lectures, American Academy of Orthopaedic Surgeons, Vol 24, 1975.

2. Lyman, HB: *Test Scores and What They Mean,* Prentice-Hall, Inc. New Jersey, 1978.

3. Bowker, AM: *Narrative Index: Standardized Assessments Used by Occupational Therapists in Physical Disabilities,* Physical Disabilities Special Interest Section Newsletter, Vol 6, No 1, 1983.

4. Strub, RL, Black, FW: *The Mental Status Examination in Neurology* F.A. Davis Co., Philadelphia, PA, 1977.

A Review of Initial Assessments Used by Occupational Therapists in Mental Health Settings

Elizabeth A. Moyer, MS, OTR, FAOTA

ABSTRACT. Factors affecting the selection and development of procedures used by occupational therapists for initial patient assessment in mental health settings are reviewed. The results of several national surveys of practicing therapists indicating those assessments most frequently taught in occupational educational programs and/or used in clinical settings are discussed. Some future trends in mental health practice are presented.

The quality of the initial assessment of patients as a basis for treatment planning is a matter of continuing concern for occupational therapists who work in mental health settings. In 1978 these therapists identified "developing, standardizing and sharing patient assessments" as the second highest 'critical issue' affecting their practice.[1] In response to this concern the American Occupational Therapy Association (AOTA) Mental Health Specialty Section (MHSS) sponsored in recent years several national surveys of practicing therapists. The results of these surveys have been used as resources in developing this paper. One of the surveys requested that therapists submit the actual assessment instruments they used. The resultant collection of instruments was screened by an MHSS committee and those tests judged most widely used or most highly developed were compiled into an index distributed by AOTA.[2] Most of the assessments reviewed were received between 1978 and 1980. Another MHSS survey of occupational therapy educators was con-

Elizabeth A. Moyer was Chairperson of the AOTA Mental Health Specialty Section 1978-80. She was former Associate Professor and Occupational Therapy Division Director at the University of Alabama in Birmingham, Alabama. At present she is a consultant in Private Practice in Tallahassee, Florida.

ducted by Hill in 1980 to ascertain the subject matter, including assessment strategies they would include in programs to update the mental health knowledge of former students.[3]

In addition to these MHSS surveys Hemphill contacted occupational therapy mental health clinicians and clinical educators as well as academic educators to determine their preferences in patient assessment.[4] In 1983 members of the AOTA Mental Health Special Interest Section expressed continuing interest in this area of practice by selecting assessment topics as the subjects most needed for continuing education.[5]

These concerns probably reflect the nation's emphasis in health care on quality assurance, accountability and cost effectiveness of services since assessment is a key to treatment effectiveness. In earlier decades many occupational therapists in mental health practice relied solely on informal methods of assessing patients' needs or depended on the evaluation information gathered by other professionals. Today occupational therapists are eager to prove the effectiveness of their services by having good baseline data for treatment planning from which subsequent progress and improvement can be measured. In addition, because of short patient stays typical today in many mental health settings assessment strategies used by occupational therapists must be brief, standardized, structured and practical. With the exception of those patients seen in state hospitals and transitional living and training programs, many persons with whom occupational therapists work now are seen for only two or three weeks. This means that without concise evaluation strategies a therapist could easily devote the entire time available for occupational therapy in assessment. In some settings in fact that is what has happened and the resultant treatment planning pertains only to community follow-up after discharge. In addition, assessment instruments used in practice must have high face validity because more educated consumers demand that evaluation and treatment relate in a direct and obvious way to their problems.

The increased demand for formalized, standard assessment tools tends to imply a devaluation by therapists of informal qualitative evaluation procedures, the use of which has been a strong characteristic of occupational therapy practice. Unfortunately, however, if informal procedures are cast aside, the occupational therapist's ability to select from a wide repertoire of evaluation tasks and to be able to assess the functioning of extremely low performing or noncommunicative patients may be lost. At the same time the waning of interest in the psychiatric community in psychodynamic treatment models and the less structured treatment approaches associated with them might prompt academic educators in the profession to discontinue the teaching of the assessment of intrapsychic processes. Besides use with low functioning psychiatric patients, the more qualitative assessments serve occupational therapists well in evaluating children and adolescents, or persons who are neurotic, traumatized, terminally ill, highly disabled physically or unable to verbalize their needs and feelings.

In recent years there has been steady growth in the numbers of behaviorally based, brief assessments and a revival of interest in prevocational programming for the psychiatric patient. Occupational therapists found little interest in the work related area of practice in the 60s and 70s, but during the practical 80s they are beginning to be drawn back to these concerns. It appears that the prevocational evaluation tools most commonly seen in use in occupational therapy clinics however have been developed by psychologists and/or work evaluators. The occupational therapist, nonetheless can offer something unique to work assessment because of his ability to conduct informal assessment of performance at tasks, to problem-solve the complex work role concerns of multiply-handicapped patients, his fundamental orientation toward task analysis and his understanding of the effects of developmental or neurological incapacity on patients' functioning. There is danger if occupational therapists indiscriminately accept available work assessments without attempting to develop and use evaluations specifically suited to the field's special talents.

Finally occupational therapists have shown an increasing interest in neurophysiological treatment models in mental health practice and this has led to a search for useful evaluation and treatment tools within the field as well as those developed by neuropsychologists and persons in related professions.

TYPES OF INITIAL ASSESSMENTS USED

Projective Tests

The projective activity battery has been the traditional assessment tool of occupational therapists in psychiatric practice for many years. Beginning with the Azima Occupational Therapy Battery,[6] the Fidler Diagnostic Battery[7] and a myriad of variations of them, occupational therapists have thrived on these assessments as basic tools for treatment planning. The batteries generally involve analysis of patient performance on several creative activities such as finger painting, clay sculpture, designing and assembling tile trivets and figure drawings. A frequent feature of such testing is a progression from structured to less structured tasks. Ordinarily use of such tests was part of the overall psychodynamic treatment model used in the treatment setting. Now surveys (already cited) have shown how assessments such as these are disappearing from occupational therapy clinics because of changes in treatment philosophies among mental health therapists. Nonetheless, as recently as 1980 Hemphill found that 87% of the occupational therapy educational programs were still teaching the Fidler assessment even though only 10% of clinicians were using it.[4]

One projective assessment, however, with growing popularity among occupational therapists is the Kinetic Family Drawing,[8] which did not originate within the profession. It taps information about family functioning as a fundamental component in today's treatment plan. Occupational therapists also frequently administer the Person Drawing.[9] This assessment can be integrated with almost any treatment model depending on how the data are interpreted and used. For example, a given drawing can be seen as an indicator of intellectual maturity,[10] developmental level of body image,[11] neurophysiological status[9] or as a simple paper-and-pencil task. Recently some projective assessments have been developed with group behaviors as a focus. Such assessments as Build-a-City by Clark[12] and Ehrenberg's Comprehensive Assessment,[13] promise a new facet to evaluation for further development in occupational therapy clinics.

The Magazine Picture Collage is the most highly developed test in terms of research with it and standardization of scoring.[14-16] This test was rapidly adopted by occupational therapists in many settings because of its low cost, ease of administration and high acceptance by adult patients.

Interviews and Questionnaires

According to data in the surveys interviewing continues to be the most common form of assessment procedure used by occupational therapists in psychiatric practice. However, efforts have been made recently to develop protocols to give more structure to interviews and even to assign ratings to patient responses. In efforts to save treatment time some therapists are asking patients to complete self-administered questionnaires which are then brought to the first therapy session for discussion and to apply in treatment planning. One of the most common questionnaires is called the Activities Configuration in which patients describe their daily activities and their feelings about those activities. Like the Person Drawing this assessment can fit into many treatment models depending on how it is interpreted. The most popular version of a questionnaire used by occupational therapists is by Watanabe[17] and variations of it continue to appear.

An instrument called 'Time Construction' is of particular interest. In it the respondent describes his daily routines concretely by pasting blocks of colored paper on a daily schedule to represent the scope and amounts of time spent in his various activities. The test was developed by Barth and Leav[18] for use with alcoholic and forensic patients. Its form lends a confrontive quality to the inquiry of the patient.

A variety of questionnaires as bases for data gathering about occupational history and role performance are associated with the occupational behavior model of treatment. One of the first to be developed was the Moorhead Occupational History Interview.[19] More recently developed assessments pertaining to this frame of reference and now adopted by many therapists are Black's Adolescent Role Assessment[20] and the Occupational Role History.[21] Occupational therapists in general have been slow to develop assessments of family relationships. One of the few available is the Bell Family Assessment,[22] a questionnaire-interview tool.

The checklist is another form of questionnaire popular in occupational therapy practice. One of the most frequently used, also related to the occupational behavior treatment model, is the Interest Check List (ICL) by Matsutsuyu.[23] It is a very flexible tool that can be adapted to a variety of treatment models. Using it patients simply check the strength of their interests in a variety of functional and recreational activities.

With the increasing interest in holistic treatment models and in prevention, more therapists are using measurements of stress and its effects to help pinpoint patient problems. One instrument of this type developed by occupational therapists, is the Stress History by Hill and Brittell.[24]

Behavioral Rating Scales

Reported as the most commonly used behavioral rating scale is the Comprehensive Occupational Therapy Evaluation Scale better known as the COTE Scale.[25] This instrument is most appropriate for use in settings with patients of short-to-medium length stays and was quickly adopted by therapists undoubtedly because it is brief, well organized and has well defined behaviors to identify. A few therapists in mental health practice have adopted one of the many functional rating scales of activities of daily living used with physically disabled patients. In addition, the Parachek Geriatric Rating Scale[26] is sometimes used for screening populations of low functioning patients.

Task Assessments

The MHSS surveys further show that task assessments are frequently used as strategies for evaluation by occupational therapists probably because of the professon's identity and basic interest in task performance. Occupational therapists in mental health, Williams and Bloomer, have developed the Bay Area Functional Performance Evaluation (BaFPE).[27] It turns out to be the instrument assessing task performance with the most research behind it, for its authors have made a concerted effort to construct and validate a reliable practice tool. The BaFPE examines the patient's functional abilities in five varied tasks. It also evaluates social interaction. In spite of fairly complex administration and scoring procedures the assessment is used in numerous clinics and is now being taught to beginning therapists in many educational programs.

The Kohlman Evaluation of Living Skills (KELS) has been even more widely adopted by therapists since its introduction in 1979.[28] This is a very basic quick assessment that seems to better fit today's needs in short-term care than any other instrument so far available. Although it is evident from reports of its use that further development of the KELS is needed, it nonetheless still stands out in popularity because of its simple and clear-cut format and highly standardized method of administration.

For use in the settings where patients stay for longer periods of time evaluations of living skills have been developed, for example, the Basic Living Skills Battery[29] and the Comprehensive Evaluation of Basic Living Skills.[30] Even though information about the Basic Living Skills Battery reached practitioners through presentation at but one AOTA Conference, it is now found in use in a number of occupational therapy programs. The Comprehensive Evaluation of Basic Living Skills, on the other hand, was published in 1976 but is still not widely used, perhaps because of its length which may require up to 8 hours to administer. Meanwhile occupational therapists are finding and using a number of useful assessments for living skills developed outside of the profession. Of particular note among them are the Street Survival Skills Questionnaire[31] from McCarron-Dial and the Independent Living Behavioral Checklist[32] developed by the West Virginia Research and Training Center.

In addition, data from the surveys show that most of the prevocational tests occupational therapists in mental health currently use have been developed outside the field. On the other hand, some therapists have used instruments which other occupational therapists have applied primarily in assessing work skills of physically disabled patients and have found them helpful. Along with occupational therapy tests of hand skills are such commonly available tests as the Bennett Hand Tool Dexterity Test, The Crawford Small Parts Dexterity Test and the MacQuarrie Test of Mechanical Ability. Principal among the major prevocational and vocational systems used in the mental health setting are those by Valpar, Singer and McCarron-Dial.

One of the most valuable contributions occupational therapists can make to work role evaluation is in physical capacities evaluation. Smith[33] has developed an excellent, relatively brief version that has become a critical factor in disability determination in the places where therapists have used it. The test should gain in importance in mental health settings as well because of the stiffening of eligibility requirements for public assistance on the basis of inability to work.

Several task-based tests of cognitive function have been developed by Allen and graduate students at the Los Angeles County/University of Southern California Medical Center. These are the Funky Pad Assembly Task,[34] the Allen Cognitive Levels[35] leather lacing and the Riska Object Classification Test[36] with cardboard shapes. As these tests become more widely available they may well be used and further tested by occupational therapists for evaluation and treatment of patients with cognitive disabilities.

Neurophysiological Assessments

The surveys show that interest is growing in mental health settings in assessments of sensory integration for both children and adult patients. Although the Ayres' Southern California Sensory Integration Tests and other developmental assessments have been available for many years, they have been used primarily with children. Therapists working with adults with suspected sensory integration deficits have been limited in evaluation to the use of non-standardized applications of parts of pediatric assessments. Available since 1979, the SBC Adult Sensory Integration Evaluation[37] is an attempt to provide to therapists in psychiatric practice a standardized test of sensory integration deficits for adult populations. Its use has improved the treatment situation for therapists and patients alike. The recently developed Warren Adult Sensory Integration Test (WASIT),[38] also for mental health settings, should be helpful once it is published. Both the SBC and the WASIT are being extensively studied especially for their abilities to separate patients with process schizophrenic profiles from normal populations. Analysis of the use with adults of some of Ayres' subtests[39, 40] may make the use of those tests more acceptable in psychiatric settings. Therapists however need to be aware of the dangers of violating the integrity of an entire battery by isolating subtests.

Therapists looking for assessments in the area of neurophysiological treatment developed by other disciplines report they have found several useful instruments. One is the Luria-Nebraska[41] which, because of its length of at least two and one-half hours to administer, has been seen in occupational therapy mainly in research studies. Psychomotility tests are also popular with the hope that such instruments may provide a quick means of screening general sensory integrative status. The Reitan Tapping Test[42] is one test that has been explored for this purpose and appears now in sensory integration batteries being tried with adults by occupational therapists. King has added to the resources available by developing norms for a very simple and inexpensive Object Manipulation Test.[43] Thus it too may soon have wider use among therapists generally.

Certain drawing tasks remain popular for detection of sensory integration dysfunction. The Person Drawing, previously noted and the Winterhaven Visual Copy Forms[44] are frequently selected for this purpose.

FUTURE DEVELOPMENTS AND CONCLUSIONS

The data from the several MHSS surveys suggest that the impetus is now strong for further development and study of the major new occupational therapy mental health tests such as the BaFPE and the

SBC, as well as on older tools like the COTE Scale and Person Drawing. The survey evidence of increased use of major 'established' assessments suggests that the proliferation of informal assessment instruments may be slowed. Therapists in mental health practice seem to have accepted the value of using recognized tests and of using standardized scoring procedures if they are to have sound data bases for treatment. This is particularly true among recent graduates who often have more training in research and in the use of statistical data than do older practitioners. As assessments developed by occupational therapists gain acceptance because of supporting research, the sifting out and refining process by users will continue. It follows then that those tests with widest use and greatest acceptance will certainly become available commercially. Increasing sensitivity to the appropriateness of particular assessments for given patient populations, treatment settings and treatment models, as well as to the need for a qualified therapist to administer them, will emerge as therapists find their treatment effectiveness enhanced by better assessment.

Assessments for use in mental health practice will undoubtedly emerge based on AOTA's endorsed Uniform Occupational Therapy Evaluation Checklist.[45] At least one such assessment is under development, the Alabama Comprehensive Occupational Therapy Screening Test.[46] In the long run the search will continue for the briefest, most discriminating tools that fit each therapist's selected philosophical model of treatment. With the growth of interest in assessment and broader study of occupational therapy evaluation tools therapists will also become more discriminating in their choices of tools developed by persons in other disciplines such as psychologists, therapists in the creative arts and vocational evaluators.

Further, the concerns of the educated consumer will continue to affect occupational therapy assessment in mental health. More tests will be reality based. More assessment strategies will be designed to be cost effective and results will be shared directly with patients. More therapists will ask patients to complete preliminary questionnaires and do self-assessments as preparation for treatment activity.

This is a time when occupational therapists in mental health practice are receptive to new developments in assessment strategies which they can use effectively. They are also becoming more sophisticated in knowing what they need and want for assessment of patients in their practice. While testing procedures that are 'old stand-bys' may be dropped because they no longer fit current treatment models, other better designed and briefer tools will replace them. The end result is that these changes should result in more effective patient treatment in occupational therapy clinics.

REFERENCES*

1. Moyer EA: Critical issues identified. *AOTA Mental Health Specialty Section Newsletter,* 2: 1, 1979.

2. Moyer EA: Index of assessments used by occupational therapists in mental health. In *Mental Health,* AOTA Division of Professional Development. Rockville, Maryland: American Occupational Therapy Association, 42-54, 1981.

3. Hill L: *Results Educator Survey 1980 Mental Health Specialty Section.* Utica, New York: Utica College.

4. Hemphill BJ: Mental health evaluations used in occupational therapy. *Am J Occup Ther* 34: 721-726, 1980.

5. Moyer EA: Continuing Education Needs of Mental Health Special Interest Section. American Occupational Therapy Association Annual Conference, Portland, April 19, 1983.

6. Azima FJ: The Azima Battery: An overview. In *The Evaluative Process in Psychiatric Occupational Therapy,* BJ Hemphill, Editor. Thorofare, New Jersey: Charles B. Slack, Inc, 57-61, 1982.

7. Fidler J & Fidler G: *Occupational Therapy: A Communicative Process in Psychiatry.* New York: MacMillan Co., 1963.

8. Burns R & Kaufman H: *Actions, Styles, and Symbols in Kinetic Family Drawings (K-F-D).* New York: Brunner/Mazel, 1972.

9. King LJ: The person symbol as an assessment tool. In *The Evaluative Process in Psychiatric Occupational Therapy,* BJ Hemphill, Editor. Thorofare, New Jersey: Charles B. Slack, Inc, 1982.

10. Harris DB: *Children's Drawings as a Measure of Intellectual Maturity.* New York: Harcourt, Brace, and World, 1963.

11. DiLeo JH: *Young Children and Their Drawings.* New York: Brunner/Mazel, 1970.

12. Dowey NL & Clark EN: "Build a City": Projective Activities in Occupational Therapy. American Occupational Therapy Association Annual Conference, San Diego, May 11, 1978.

13. Ehrenberg F: Comprehensive assessment process: A group evaluation. In *The Evaluative Process in Psychiatric Occupational Therapy,* BJ Hemphill, Editor. Thorofare, New Jersey: Charles B. Slack, Inc, 155-167, 1982.

14. Buck R & Provancher MA: Magazine picture collages as an evaluation technique. *Am J Occup Ther* 26: 36-39, 1972.

15. Lerner C: The magazine picture collage: Its clinical use and validity as an assessment device. *Am J Occup Ther* 33: 500-504, 1979.

16. Lerner C: The magazine picture collage. In *The Evaluative Process in Psychiatric Occupational Therapy,* BJ Hemphill, Editor. Thorofare, New Jersey: Charles B. Slack, Inc, 139-154, 1982.

17. Watanabe S: Social adaptation: "Making it." In the *1968 AOTA Regional Institutes on the Evaluation Process, Final Report,* RSA 123-T-68.

18. Barth T & Leav W: *Time Construction.* New York, New York: St. Vincent's Hospital, 1978.

19. Moorehead L: The occupational history, *Am J Occup Ther* 23: 329-334, 1969.

20. Black M: Adolescent role assessment. *Am J Occup Ther* 30: 73-79, 1976.

---

*Some reference listings appear as incomplete. These merely reflect information given in survey responses.

21. Florey L & Michelman S: Occupational role history: A screening tool for psychiatric occupational therapy. *Am J Occup Ther* 36, 301-308, 1982.

22. Bell J: *The Bell Family Assessment Inventory.*

23. Matsutsuyu J: The interest check list. *Am J Occup Ther* 23, 323-328, 1969.

24. Hill L & Brittell T: *Stress History Outline,* Utica, New York: Utica College, 1981.

25. Brayman SJ, Kirby TF, Misenheimer AM & Short MJ: Comprehensive occupational therapy evaluation scale. *Am J Occup Ther* 30, 94-100, 1976.

26. Parachek JF & King LJ: *Parachek Geriatric Rating Scale and Treatment Manual.* Phoenix: Center for Neurodevelopmental Studies, Inc, 1982.

27. Bloomer JS & Williams SK: *Bay Area Functional Performance Evaluation (Research Edition).* Palo Alto, California: Consulting Psychologists, Inc, 1980.

28. McGourty LK: *Kohlman Evaluation of Living Skills (KELS): Interim Manual.* Seattle, 1979.

29. Chapman-Broekema M & Skolaski T: An Assessment Tool for Community Psychiatric Treatment: The Basic Living Skills Battery. American Occupational Therapy Association Annual Conference, Milwaukee, October 16, 1975.

30. Casanova JS & Ferber J: Comprehensive evaluation of basic living skills. *Am J Occup Ther* 30: 143-47, 1976.

31. Linkenhoker D & McCarron L: *Adaptive Behavior: Street Survival Skills Questionnaire.* Dallas: McCarron-Dial Systems, 1979.

32. Walls RT, Zane T & Thvedt JE: *Independent Living Behavioral Checklist.* Dunbar, West Virginia: West Virginia Research and Training Center.

33. Smith SL: The physical capacities evaluation. In *Willard and Spackman's Occupational Therapy,* 6th Edition, HL Hopkins and HD Smith, Editors. Philadelphia: J. B. Lippincott, 168-173, 1983.

34. Herzig S: *Occupational Therapy Assessment of Cognitive Levels as Predictors of Community Adjustment of Chronic Schizophrenia Patients.* Thesis, University of Southern California, 1978.

35. Moore D: *An Occupational Therapy Evaluation of Sensorimotor Cognition: Initial Reliability, Validity, and Descriptive Data for Hospitalized Schizophrenic Adults.* Thesis, University of Southern California, 1978.

36. Williams LR: *Development and Initial Testing of an Occupational Therapy Object Classification Test.* Thesis, University of Southern California, 1981.

37. Schroeder CV, Block MP, Trottier EC & Stowell MS: The adult psychiatric sensory integrative evaluation. In *The Evaluative Process in Psychiatric Occupational Therapy,* BJ Hemphill, Editor. Thorofare, New Jersey: Charles B. Slack, Inc, 1982.

38. Pettit KA & Utley ER: Evaluating and Treating Depressed Vestibular Processing in Chronic Psychiatric Patients. American Occupational Therapy Association Annual Conference, Philadelphia, May 11, 1982.

39. Hsu YT & Nelson DL: Adult performance on the Southern California Kenesthesis and Tactile Perception Tests. *Am J Occup Ther* 35: 788-791, 1981.

40. Petersen P & Wikoff RL: The performance of adult males on the Southern California Figure-Ground Visual Perception Test. *Am J Occup Ther* 37: 554-560, 1983.

41. Golden CJ, Hammeke TA & Purisch AD: *Luria-Nebraska Neuropsychological Battery, Manual.* Los Angeles: Western Psychological Services.

42. Reitan RM: *Manual for Administration of Neuropsychological Test Batteries for Adults and Children.* Indianapolis: Indiana University Medical Center.

43. King LJ: *The Object Manipulation Speed Test.* Scottsdale, Arizona: Greenroom Publications, 1978.

44. King LJ: *Winter Haven Scoring Sheet.* Phoenix: Arizona State Hospital. (For a version adapted for adults, ages 18-40).

45. Hopkins HL & Smith HD: *Willard and Spackman's Occupational Therapy,* 6th Edition. Philadelphia: J.B. Lippincott, 1983.

46. Division of Occupational Therapy 1982 Senior Class: *Alabama Comprehensive Occupational Therapy Screening (ALCOTS), Therapist Instruction Manual.* Birmingham: University of Alabama in Birmingham, 1981.

Identifying Leisure Interests: A Self-Assessment Approach for Adults With Arthritis

Lisette N. Kautzmann, MS, OTR

ABSTRACT. Helping adults learn to live with arthritis is a major responsibility of occupational therapists. There are a variety of instruments for therapists to use in evaluating the self-care and work components of occupational performance, however there are no instruments for assessing the leisure interests of persons with arthritis. The purpose of this investigation was to develop an instrument for assessing the leisure interests of adults with rheumatoid arthritis or degenerative joint disease. The instrument is patterned after Knowles self-diagnostic competency model.

Following Knowles' procedure of developing such a model, a literature review and a panel of occupational therapists with expertise in the treatment of rheumatic disease were used to identify a list of leisure activities. The list was categorized and applied to Knowles' suggested format for a self-diagnostic competency model. Strategies for using the instrument with the targeted population are presented.

Adults with rheumatoid arthritis or degenerative joint disease often are required to modify their life styles as a result of the disease process. The resulting curtailment of activity may have far reaching effects. Individuals with arthritis often report feelings of helplessness, dependency, and confinement. Inclusion of the leisure component of occupational performance in the assessment and treatment of adults with arthritis is vital to their eventual adjustment to life style

Lisette N. Kautzmann is Academic Fieldwork Coordinator, Occupational Therapy Program, School of Allied Health Professions, University of Wisconsin-Milwaukee, Milwaukee, WI 53201.

The author would like to extend thanks to Lynn Caruso, MS, OTR, and the staff of the Occupational Therapy Department, Columbia Hospital, Milwaukee, WI, for reviewing the list of activities. This research was conducted in partial fulfillment of the requirements for a Doctor of Education degree at Nova University.

For a copy of the self-assessment instrument, please write Lisette Kautzmann, Occupational Therapy Program, University of Wisconsin-Milwaukee, PO Box 413, Milwaukee, WI 53201.

changes. It also is a legitimate concern of the holistic occupational therapist.

Leisure is the area of occupational performance that preserves and promotes linkages between individuals with arthritis, other people and the community. These linkages serve to prevent the spiral of isolation, decreased self-worth and depression that can assail persons with arthritis as they struggle to cope with the disease process and life style change. Encouraging the development of leisure interests that are within the capabilities of adults with rheumatic disease helps them cope with a chronic disability and the restrictions it places on their life style, since many individuals are discouraged by their inability to participate in their usual work, self-care and leisure activities.[1]

Although occupational therapists are concerned with evaluating all three occupational performance components, the area of leisure assessment has not received as much attention as evaluation of self-care skills and vocational assessment. Several instruments have been developed to assess the self-care and work skills of adults with arthritis;[1] however, the problem is that there are no instruments for occupational therapists to use in assessing the leisure interests of this population. The purpose of this investigation was to develop a leisure interest self-assessment instrument based on Knowle's self-diagnostic competency model, for occupational therapists to use in treatment planning with their adult arthritic clients.

Two criteria were established for the design of the self-assessment instrument. The first criterion was that the instrument should include activities which generally do not contribute to joint damage or fatigue in adults with rheumatoid arthritis or degenerative joint disease. The second criterion was that the instrument should allow the respondents to actively participate in the self-diagnosis of their needs and interests. Since a majority of the persons diagnosed as having rheumatoid arthritis or degenerative joint disease are adults, it seemed appropriate to use an adult education competency model for self-diagnosing learning needs as the format for the leisure assessment instrument.

LITERATURE REVIEW

Although much has been written about evaluating the self-care and work components of occupational performance,[1-5] very little has appeared in the occupational therapy literature regarding leisure assessment. The major investigation in this area of occupational performance was reported by Matsutsuyu in 1969.[6] Matsutsuyu's instrument, the Neuropsychiatric Institute (NPI) Interest Check List, was developed for a psychiatric population. It allows classification of the intensity and types of interest for each of the 80 listed items, description of the individual's ability to express personal preference, and delineation of the individual's capacity to discriminate type and intensity. The activities listed are limited to those which could be carried out within the NPI Occupational Therapy Department. Matsutsuyu suggests that further information and clarification may be obtained through a follow-up interview.

In reviewing the therapeutic recreation literature, several of the instruments designed to assess leisure interests in normal and handicapped populations were identified. A survey of the most frequently used leisure assessments for people with normal intelligence[7] indicated that all of the instruments are self-reports and require professional scoring and interpretation.

An examination of the vocational rehabilitation literature reveals an Avocational Activities Inventory developed by Owens[8] that is a systematic classification of avocational activities. In addition to listing general types of avocational activities, an effort was made to include in the inventory activities for elderly and severely disabled people. Owens divides avocational activities into nine major categories with specific activities listed under each category.

Knowles provides a comprehensive overview of adult education philosophy and methodology.[9] In describing facilitators of adult learning, Knowles states that truly artistic teachers of adults perceive the locus of responsibility for learning to be within the learner. According to Knowles, the use of a self-diagnostic competency model is the newest approach to helping adults assume responsibility for assessing their learning needs. Knowles suggests that a competency model may be developed in one of the following ways: a review of the existing literature, the judgement of experts regarding the required competencies for performing a desired role, through task analysis by observation of the competencies possessed by the most effective performers, and through group participation in model building. The resulting list of activities or competencies is then applied to a format, described by Knowles, which consists of three categories of response for each item on the list. The first category of response is importance to my career, the second category is importance to my self-actualization, and the third category is level of participation. Under each of these major category headings are subcategories of none, medium and high.

METHODS

In developing the self-assessment instrument, leisure activities that generally do not contribute to joint-damage and fatigue in people with either rheumatoid arthritis or degenerative joint disease were identified, organized and incorporated into the suggested format of Knowles' self-diagnostic competency model. Using Knowles' recommended procedure for developing a competency model, a list of leisure activities was identified through a review of the literature in occupational therapy, therapeutic recreation, and vocational rehabilitation. The list was screened to eliminate activities that consistently would contribute to joint damage and fatigue. The screened list of activities was then submitted to a panel of occupational therapists who are knowledgeable in the treatment of rheumatic disease for review and recommendations regarding the appropriateness of each listed activity for the targeted population. A modification of Owen's Avocational Activities Inventory was used to categorize the finalized list of activities. The categorized list of leisure activities was applied to Knowles' self-diagnostic competency model format.

Content validity is assumed on the basis of the representative sampling of activities from the literature review, the screening process and the agreement of the panel of reviewers on the appropriateness of each item for the targeted population. Since this instrument was designed to facilitate the self-diagnosis of leisure interests of the individual adult, no attempt has been made to establish norms for the instrument. Instrument reliability may be affected by the respondent's mood, energy level and pain.

RESULTS

The finalized list of leisure activities consists of 64 items (see Table 1). Using a modification of Owen's Avocational Activities Inventory, these 64 items were placed in one of the following categories: games, sports and movement activities, creative arts and crafts, entertainment, organization activities and educational activi-

Table 1

Walking	Dramatics	Attending concerts	Board games
Bicycling	Traveling	Collecting coins	Card games
Swimming	Dining-out	Collecting stamps	Viewing sporting events
Boating	Shopping	Collecting guns	Relaxation exercises
Camping	Tobaggoning	Collecting rocks & minerals	T'ai Chi Ch'uan
Fishing	Nature walks	Collecting/gathering shells	Observing nature
Gardening	Flower arranging	Collecting antiques	Religious activites
Cooking	Flower drying/pressing	Collecting dolls	PTA & school activities
Winemaking	Model building	Collecting figurines	Social club activities
Sewing	Listening to music	Collecting china & glass	Civic activities
Ceramics	Creative writing	Playing video games	Political activities
Painting	Watching T.V.	Completing puzzles	Informational lectures
Singing	Caring for pets	Playing minature golf	"How-to" courses
Reading	Entertaining	Playing croquet	Self-improvement courses
Photography	Creative stitching	Playing badminton	Attending academic courses
	Caring for houseplants	Playing a musical instrument	Visiting friends/relatives

ties. An additional item of "other" was added at the end of each category to accommodate special interest areas.

At the recommendation of the review panel, the column headings suggested by Knowles were revised to read: importance of this activity to me, my present level of skill or interest and my priorities for further development and participation. Under each column heading are sub-columns of none, low, medium and high.

The instrument is organized as a grid with the activities listed vertically and the column and sub-column headings arranged horizontally. The only materials required to complete the self-assessment are a pen or pencil. Participants are asked to indicate a response to each listed activity. The items that receive a rating of high in the column headed "my priorities for future development and participation" provide the focus for action and treatment planning.

DISCUSSION

The two pre-established criteria were met in the following manner. The needs of the targeted population were addressed through the list of activities specifically designed for adults with arthritis. The use of the competency model as the structural format allows the respondents to actively participate in the self-diagnosis of their needs and interests. The instrument is performance-oriented and self-scoring, which gives the respondents immediate feedback and a focus for future action. It also serves as a vehicle for facilitating further discussion of leisure interests and treatment planning.

The self-assessment instrument has been well received by persons with arthritis and used effectively in a variety of settings. Adults with arthritis report that they are encouraged by the wide range of listed activities and the focus on engagement rather than curtailment of activity. Therapists have used the self-assessment instrument with individuals, small groups, and general audiences of up to 160 adults. The recommended procedure in all situations is a two-step process of allowing the respondent(s) to complete the self-assessment, followed by a discussion of the results and identification of community resources. A list of community facilities is a helpful adjunct to this discussion. Whenever possible, individuals with arthritis should be encouraged to participate in activities that are designed for the general public, because these activities offer a diversity that is not present when participation is limited to programs for the handicapped.

An effective strategy for managing large groups is to provide one discussion group for each major category of leisure interest with a knowledgeable person assigned to each group to act as a facilitator. Participants use the results of the self-assessment to select an appropriate group and the discussion for networking and information sharing. Further discussion with the individual's occupational therapist or physician is recommended, because although the listed activities generally are appropriate for people with rheumatoid arthritis and degenerative joint disease not all activities are appropriate for every person at each stage of his or her disease. However, once a focus of interest has been established, occupational therapists usually are able to use the treatment planning discussion to suggest a modification, adaptation or a related activity if the identified leisure interest is contraindicated.

SUMMARY

The rationale and procedure for development of a leisure interest self-assessment instrument for adults with rheumatoid arthritis or degenerative joint disease were described. Strategies for using the instrument with the targeted population were discussed. The self-assessment instrument provides occupational therapists with a means of examining the leisure component of occupational performance and serves as a vehicle for facilitating a change in life style for adults with arthritis that supports and strengthens links with others and with the community.

REFERENCES

1. Melvin JL: *Rheumatic Disease: Occupational Therapy and Rehabilitation,* 2nd Edition. Philadelphia: F.A. Davis, 297-313, 1982.

2. Casanova JS, Ferber J: Comprehensive Evaluation of Basic Living Skills. *Am J Occup Ther* 30: 101-105, 1976.

3. Kester DL: Prevocational and Vocational Assessment. In *Willard and Spackman's Occupational Therapy,* 5th Edition, HL Hopkins, HD Smith Editors. Philadelphia: Lippincott, 203-218, 1978.

4. Malick, MH, Sherry B: Activities of Daily Living and Homemaking. In *Willard and Spackman's Occupational Therapy,* 5th Edition, HL Hopkins, HD Smith Editors. Philadelphia: Lippincott, 184-202, 1978.

5. Pedretti LW: *Occupational Therapy: Practice Skills for Physical Dysfunction.* St. Louis: Mosby, 64-81, 1981.

6. Matsutsuyu JS: The Interest Check List. *Am J Occup Ther* 23: 323-328, 1969.

7. Walshe WA: Avocational Counseling Interests. In *Perspectives on Leisure Counsel-*

ing, DM Compton, JE Goldstein Editors. Arlington, VA: National Recreation and Park Association, 107-119, 1977.

8. Owens RP: *Avocational Activities Inventory*. Milwaukee, WI: Curative Workshop of Milwaukee, 8-37, 1971.

9. Knowles MS: *The Modern Practice of Adult Education*. Chicago: Follett, 227-229, 1980.

Occupational Therapy Assessment and Treatment in a Hospital Setting for Patients with Epilepsy

Stephanie Day, MA, OTR

ABSTRACT. One Reed is a unit at the UCLA Neuropsychiatric Institute for the evaluation and treatment of patients with poorly controlled seizure disorders. Like many other patients with epilepsy, these individuals frequently experience problems in many facets of daily living. This paper describes the twofold purpose of occupational therapy on One Reed: to provide a program of activity and socialization during the extended period of medical evaluation, and to help patients identify problems in their daily life activities and develop the skills which will enable them to function better after hospitalization.

The frame of reference which guides practice is identified and the methods and instruments of occupational therapy assessment for this patient population are described. Typical examples of daily living problems are given, and some occupational therapy methods for dealing with the problems are enumerated.

INTRODUCTION

One Reed is a six-bed unit within the University of California at Los Angeles (UCLA) Neuropsychiatric Institute (NPI) whose patients have seizure disorders which have remained poorly controlled despite reasonable medical treatment. Patients range in age from early childhood through adulthood, and come from many parts of the country. They are admitted for two to four weeks of 24-hour per day seizure monitoring, the behavioral aspect observed by closed circuit TV and the electrical component (brain waves) by telemetry electroencephalography (EEG). The purpose of monitoring is: 1) to

---

Stephanie Day is a Senior Occupational Therapist, University of California at Los Angeles, Neuropsychiatric Institute, 760 Westwood Plaza, Los Angeles, CA 90024.

confirm or deny a diagnosis of epilepsy (ruling out pseudo or hysterical seizures) and to plan appropriate treatment, 2) to diagnose seizure type(s) and adjust anticonvulsant medications accordingly or 3) to evaluate the patient for surgical treatment. Recurrent seizures are the only medical problem for some patients, while others have a combination of difficulties ranging from subtle deficits in learning and personality to cerebral palsy or mental retardation.

Like many persons with epilepsy, One Reed patients often experience problems with daily living. As the Committee for the Control of Epilepsy and its Consequences stated, "The social, psychological and behavioral problems that frequently accompany epilepsy can be more handicapping than the actual seizures."[1] Beginning in childhood, the person with recurrent seizures may have problems in school performance, in play activities, or in relationships with peers and family members. In adolescence these difficulties may be compounded and the youth with epilepsy may fall behind in developing responsibility for himself, independence from his parents, in having meaningful relationships with the opposite sex and in developing interests, habits, skills and values for future work (the occupational choice process). The adult with chronic seizures may have deficits in daily living skills, problems in obtaining and maintaining work and in having satisfying leisure activities and socialization.[1-5]

The remainder of this paper will describe the purpose of occupational therapy on One Reed and the process and instruments used in assessment. Examples of typical problems identified and activities used to address the problems will also be given.

THE PURPOSE OF OCCUPATIONAL THERAPY ON ONE REED

The purpose of occupational therapy on One Reed is twofold. First, as the process of medical evaluation through seizure monitoring means a period of boredom and isolation for the patient, occupational therapy provides a program of activities and socialization during hospitalization appropriate for each patient's developmental level, interests and capabilities. Many patients also report that in their daily lives they lack or function poorly in "occupation" i.e., satisfying, purposeful activity, whether this be in work, leisure or activities of daily living. Secondly, then, the occupational therapy program helps patients to identify problems in daily living and to develop the skills they need to function better when they leave the hospital. In addition, the therapist works with patients to identify and adapt daily living patterns that may affect the frequency and severity of their seizures or their safety and well-being when seizures do occur.

THE EVALUATION PROCESS

As the age range of One Reed patients is wide and their needs are varied, the Occupational Behavior frame of reference is used to guide practice, because it provides a view of the "entire developmental continuum of work and play."[6] The frame of reference is built around the concepts of patient achievement, play and work, and role,[7] and helps delineate the assessment of the individual patient's needs for occupational therapy. A combination of methods for clinical data collection which is common to occupational therapy in general[8] and to Occupational Behavior in particular is employed, i.e., questionnaires, interview and observation of patients in activities. Using these methods, age-appropriate evaluation is performed for all patients. However, due to length limitations in this article and because the majority of One Reed patients are young adults, only the process for evaluating adults will be discussed here.

On the day of admission, each patient is met by the therapist and the twofold purpose of occupational therapy on the unit is explained. The patient is asked to complete the NPI Interest Checklist and a questionnaire developed on One Reed called the Occupational and Leisure Assessment for Adults with Epilepsy (OLAAE). Following a review of his responses, an interview is done and the individual occupational therapy program planned. Observations of the patient's performance are made during all activities. The evaluation information is shared with other staff members through patient charts and weekly staff meetings. Each of the assessment procedures will be explained in subsequent sections.

The NPI Interest Checklist

The NPI Interest Checklist (ICL)[9] is used to assess the patient's interest in activities. A patient's responses describe his capacity to discriminate and to express his personal preference and classify type and intensity of interest in various activities. The ICL is used as a basis on which to plan activities during the patient's stay in the hospital and/or to build a more satisfying repertoire of activities following hospitalization.

The Questionnaire

In occupational therapy, questionnaires are used to collect data from patients in nearly all diagnostic categories and from within almost all models of practice.[7] Such a questionnaire used here is the Occupational and Leisure Assessment for Adults with Epilepsy (OLAAE).* It is organized around the Occupational Behavior concepts of occupational role and the skills and habits necessary to support competent function, originally delineated by Moorehead in her work on occupational role.[10] It has evolved over time in response to increasing knowledge of the daily living situations of people with chronic seizures, and is used to identify strengths and problems in all areas of daily living. Each patient is asked to complete the questionnaire independently. If the patient is unable to do so (due, for example, to visual, motor or cognitive deficits), the therapist uses the questionnaire to structure an interview to collect the desired information. Where necessary, the patient's responses may be reviewed with family members for confirmation or clarification.

The OLAEE is divided into five basic parts: identifying data, occupational role function, daily living skills, leisure and social function and miscellaneous. Each section is described below.

Section I. Identifying Data: This section provides basic information about the individual, i.e., name, birthdate, address and type and amount of education completed. Questions regarding the type and frequency of seizures are also included here. Information from this section indicates a general level at which the person may be functioning and how much interference with daily life tasks seizures may be causing.

Section II, Occupational Role Performance: This section is divided into four parts corresponding to the four adult occupational roles identified in the Occupational Behavior frame of reference for treatment—student, worker, homemaker and retiree. Patients who do regular volunteer work are asked to complete the "worker" section. Questions within each part are designed to collect some history of the person within that role and identify competencies and prob-

---

*Copies of OLAAE are available upon request from the author.

lems in it. The individual's satisfaction within the role and/or desire for change are also examined. Questions specifically related to the effect of seizures on role performance are included in each part. Figure 1 illustrates this section with questions regarding the worker role.

Section III, Daily Living Skills: The third section covers general daily living skills, i.e., the patient's current living situation, household management, money management and community mobility. It is designed to identify strengths and problems encountered in general tasks of daily living which may or may not be directly related to the occurrence of seizures. Information is sought on actual performance, the effects of seizures on performance and/or desire for change. Figure 2 shows the type of information (on community mobility) sought in this section.

Section IV, Leisure, Socialization and Time Management: The leisure subsection asks the patient to identify hobby and leisure activities, frequency of participation, satisfaction or difficulty with activ-

Figure 1

Occupational and Leisure Assessment for Adults with Epilspsy (OLAAE)
(Worker Role Section)

Worker Role

Do you work now? yes ___ no___ If yes, what is your job? ____ If no, have you ever worked? ____ How recently? ____ Longest job held (type of job) ____ Dates of employment ____ What was your favorite job? ____ Why? ____ If unemployed, why did you leave work? ____ Would you like to work again? yes___ no ___ uncertain ____ Have you had problems related to job task? ____ job satisfaction? ___ co-workers? ___ supervisors? ____ absences? ____ seizures at work? ____ injuries? ____ other? (explain) ____ If employed: Are you satisfied with your current work? Very? ___ Moderately ____ Not at all____ Unsure ____ Do you want to make a career change? yes ___ no ___ What have you considered? ____ Do you need additional skills? yes ___ no ____ Would occupational counseling be helpful? yes ____ no ____

ities and whether and how seizures affect participation. The socialization subsection identifies friends, relatives and social groups with whom the patient is in contact, the frequency of contact, satisfaction with social outlets and whether and how epilepsy has affected this area of function. In the time management subsection, the patient estimates the amount of free time he has per week, how it is used and whether it is satisfactory. A report of a typical weekday and weekend are also requested. Problems and/or desire for change are identified. Figure 3 gives questions from the leisure section of the questionnaire.

Figure 2

Occupational and Leisure Assessment for Adults with Epilepsy (OLAAE)

(Portion of Daily Living Skills Section)

Community Mobility

For transportation do you use? Public transportation ____ Own transportation ____ Rely on others ____ Is this a problem for you? _____ In what ways? ____ Do you have trouble finding places? yes ____ no ____ sometimes ____ Do you become lost easily? yes ____ no ____ sometimes ____ Do you do better with verbal/written instructions or with maps/diagrams? ____

Figure 3

Occupational and Leisure Assessment for Adults with Epilepsy (OLAAE)

(Leisure Section)

Leisure

Do you engage in hobbies or in leisure interest activities? not at all ____ regularly ____ occasionally ____ If so, describe them. _______ What do you do for entertainment? _____ What do you do for relaxation? _____ Are you satisfied with your leisure activities? yes____ no ____ if not, what new leisure interests would you like to develop? _____ Do your seizures affect your participation? ______ How? ______ Do you need information on community resources for leisure activities? _______

Section V. Miscellaneous: This section is intended to deal with miscellaneous factors (such as stress) related to the occurrence of seizures. It also examines brain functions (such as memory) commonly associated with seizures that are apt to cause difficulty in performance in daily life.

The Interview

An interview is used for verification and clarification of the patient's responses to the questionnaire or to gather additional information. It is also used as an opportunity to collaborate with the patient in identification of problems which occupational therapy can address and to plan the specific program.

Observation

Because problems in school and work are common with patients with epilepsy, it is important for the therapist to identify whether deficits in task performance contribute to these problems. During occupational therapy, observation is made of the patient's manual skills, attention span, decision-making and problem-solving abilities, capacity to learn and retain information, to use resources, to set and implement goals and the quality of his work. Ability to structure time around tasks, to work with others, take direction or supervision and self evaluation of work are also noted and considered important dimensions of function. When problems in socialization have been identified through the questionnaire, observation of patients during group activities may be helpful in understanding such difficulties.

ASSESSMENT AND CORRESPONDING OCCUPATIONAL THERAPY

Although space does not allow reporting of many examples, a typical response from each section of the OLAAE will be given to demonstrate how the information is used by the therapist. Some examples will show also how questionnaire information may need clarification or elaboration in interview and observation.

Section I, Identifying Data; Education: "How much education have you completed?" LB reported that he had earned a B.A. in theater arts. He worked as an extra in TV and the movies, but was dissatisfied and wanted to progress to spoken parts. In interview, he reported that he had obtained his degree nine years earlier but had subsequently been ineffective in furthering his career. His present level of functioning was lower than expected for a college graduate, but observation in tasks revealed some contributing factors. He had difficulty with memory, decision making, problem solving and goal setting and implementation. In occupational therapy, some sessions were used for him to practice these capacities in the context of craft activities. In other sessions, his career goals were examined and alternatives sought. A community referral was made to help him with his career after hospitalization, and he made an appointment with the agency before leaving. To aid his poor memory, an appointment book was initiated for him to record his appointments and a tentative list of subjects to be discussed in interviews was written. He was encouraged to keep "minutes" of his appointments and to write down "assignments" from them.

Section II: Occupational Role Performance; Student Role: "Has epilepsy caused problems for you in the student role? If yes, what kinds of problems?" DH stated that he had problems as a student—with memory, frequent absences, transportation and anxiety that he would have a seizure in class. In interview, he reported that he was soon returning to school to get his General Equivalency Diploma (GED), while observation of his task performance revealed that he had never developed adequate habits to support the student role. He forgot assignments, had difficulty structuring his time and tasks and neglected to ask for help when he did not understand. In occupational therapy, craft activities were used to help him develop some of these habits. He was asked to structure his time by making a week's written schedule, including an hour a day for work on a craft of his choice. Instructions for projects were given step by step, both in writing and in verbal-demonstration combination. Once he understood a process, he was asked to work independently but to ask for help if he got "stuck." At project completion, he was asked to evaluate his work and was given feedback on it.

Section III: Daily Living Skills; Household Management: "Do you do your own cooking—regularly, rely on others, eat out, varies?" "Do you have problems with—meal planning, preparation, shopping?" PP either ate out or relied on his mother for meals. Eating out was becoming too expensive, and his working mother was unhappy with his need for her support. He identified problems in meal planning, preparation and shopping. He was included in weekly groups for meal planning and preparation, to learn basic principles of nutrition and kitchen safety and the beginning skills in planning and preparation of meals. He was put "in charge" of the shopping list to help him improve his organizational skills. A conference was held with his mother regarding his need to practice these skills and a class in basic cooking at a community college near his home was recommended.

Section IV: Leisure, Socialization and Time Management; Socialization: "Do you have good friends—many, several, few, one, none?" "Relatives?" (same categories) "How often do you get together with them?" KK indicated that she had few friends and got together with peers rarely. Because her parents were worried about her safety, she spent most of her time at home and felt lonely and isolated. Regular occupational therapy group activities were used to provide opportunities for socialization while in the hospital, and she and her family worked with the therapist to improve her opportunities for socialization following her return home. Her church was found to have both group and individual activities which she could attend. Her family believed she would be safe there, and agreed to take her more often.

Section V: Miscellaneous; Stress: "Are your seizures worse or more frequent when you are under stress?" "What kinds of things are stressful for you?" WP stated that his seizures were worse when he was stressed, and that financial matters, staying home every day and "not being occupied" were all stressful for him. While in the hospital, he was able to structure his time provided activities in which he was interested were available, but he needed direction in finding activities outside the hospital. He was encouraged to undertake a volunteer position at the hospital after discharge, and at last report, he and his girlfriend were both volunteering regularly. They reported that they now had fewer financial worries, as they had something to do "besides spending money."

CONCLUSION

This paper has reviewed occupational therapy evaluation and treatment in a hospital setting for persons with poorly controlled seizures. The methods and process of evaluation were reviewed, some typical problems in daily living identified and occupational therapy's efforts at remediation given. In some cases, work with families or referral to community agencies after hospitalization are mentioned. These functions are an important part of the therapist's role in this setting, as the hospital can provide for the patient only the beginnings of change in skills and habits needed to support competent and satisfying function in roles of daily life. Family and community support for the maintenance and further development of such skills and habits is urgent if the person with epilepsy is to attain desired goals. In this followup facet of patient care, the occupational therapist collaborates with the physicians, nurses and social workers to make discharge plans for home programs, aftercare or community placement as needed.

Although patients with seizure disorders are frequently seen in occupational therapy clinics, there seems to be little evidence from the professional literature to date that our discipline has addressed epilepsy except as a secondary diagnosis. It is suggested here that occupational therapy can be valuable in helping the patient with epilepsy to cope better with some of his daily living problems. The Occupational Behavior approach to assessment and treatment can provide bases on which the therapist organizes a program to address the special problems in daily life activities and socialization faced by people with epilepsy.

REFERENCES

1. Sands, HE, Editor: *Epilepsy, A Handbook for the Mental Health Professional,* NY: Bruner/Mazel, 1982, p xi.

2. Svoboda, WB: *Learning About Epilepsy,* Baltimore: University Park Press, 1979.

3. Hermann, BP, Editor: *A Multidisciplinary Handbook of Epilepsy,* Springfield, Ill: Charles C Thomas, 1980.

4. Sullivan, MW: *Living With Epilepsy,* Modesto, CA: Bubba Press, 1981.

5. Day, SM: OT program development within a hospital setting for patients with epilepsy, *AOTA DDSIS Newsletter,* Vol. 5, #1: 1-2, 1982.

6. Matsutsuyu, J: Occupational behavior, a perspective on work and play, *Am J Occup Ther* 25: 291-294, 1971, 1971, p 291.

7. Matsutsuyu, J: Occupational behavior approach, *Willard and Spackman's Occupational Therapy,* 6th ed, HL Hopkins, HD Smith, Editors, Philadelphia: JB Lippincott, 1983.

8. Hemphill, B, Editor: *The Evaluative Process in Psychiatric Occupational Therapy,* Thorofare, NJ: Charles B Slack, 1982.

9. Matsutsuyu, J: The interest checklist, *Am J Occup Ther* 23: 319-322, 1969.

10. Moorehead, L: The occupational history, *Am J Occup Ther* 23: 329-334, 1969.

Assessment of the Hemiparetic Upper Extremity: A Functional Test

Dorothy J. Wilson, BS, OTR, FAOTA

ABSTRACT. The Functional Test gives an accurate and immediate assessment of upper extremity capabilities for performance of functional activities. It has been used primarily with patients who have a residual hemiparetic upper extremity following a stroke. This seventeen task test is arranged in seven levels and can be administered in approximately thirty minutes. It is completely portable and can be used practically in many different treatment settings. The information obtained will allow therapists to set realistic functional goals and design effective programs for the patient's use of the involved upper extremity. The early research on this instrument implies that this test may be used as an alternative to some of the traditional objective and time consuming test measures that are currently used by occupational therapists.

INTRODUCTION

This Functional Test was developed for use with patients who have residual neurological deficits in the involved upper extremity following a cerebral vascular accident. The need for such an assessment tool that provides reliable data and permits completion in a brief amount of time is easily understood. The recent development of prospective payment plans and their impact on practice and the ever shrinking amounts of time that are authorized for treatment

---

Dorothy J. Wilson is Director of Occupational Therapy at Rancho Los Amigos Hospital, 7601 East Imperial Highway, Downey, California 90242. Dorothy is an active member of AOTA, AOTPAC, WFOT, OTAC and CFOT and is the immediate past chair of the AOTA Physical Disabilities Special Interest Section.

Thanks to Lucinda Baker, PT, and Judy Craddock, OTR, who assisted with the development of this test. The test was developed during a study that was supported, in part, by the Veteran's Administration, contract V101 (134) P545.

forces the therapist to find the most cost effective and efficient assessment and treatment methods available.

The most useful tests are those which provide data that enables the therapist to plan effective treatment to improve the patient's functional status. If the test also objectively measures the improvement in the patient's ability during the treatment process, its value to the therapist is increased.

This article describes a test that assesses the patient's overall motor capability for upper extremity function in terms that are easily reported and easily translated into therapeutic goals.

TRADITIONAL ASSESSMENT

Many assessments of the hemiparetic upper extremity carefully dissect the separate neurological components that impact on function. The occupational therapist commonly uses a battery of tests that may include goniometric joint range measurements to determine limitations in motion; dynamometric readings of voluntary grasp; sensory testing and other assessments of the quantity and quality of voluntary and involuntary motor control. The latter includes the patient's ability to open the hand for grasp. Current patterns of testing motor control generally employ an eclectic combination of methods that is most comfortable for the particular therapist.[1, 2] The findings of the motor assessment are usually described in terms of presence or absence of synergies, motions deviating from synergies and isolated muscle function. Some attempts are made to rate the presence of excessive tone or spasticity and of sensory impairments and their influence on function. In addition, most commonly used assessments include descriptive ratings of cognitive and perceptual abilities.

After administering these isolated tests, the therapist must then put the dissected pieces together in a manner that will accurately reflect the functional capability of the hemiparetic upper extremity. This integration is frequently a difficult task for new and inexperienced therapists. The data collected on the separate tests and measures is meaningless unless the therapist is able to synthesize and summarize the information in a way that gives a clear and concise picture of the patient's ability to use the hemiparetic upper extremity. Skill in interpreting the significance of joint contractures, motor control deficits, sensory impairments, or cognitive limitations is based on the therapist's understanding of how these deficits impact on function.

Since the major problem with this approach to assessment is the difficulty in integrating the parts into a meaningful whole, what is needed is a tool that can directly assess functional capability. To be practical for the occupational therapist, such an assessment should be able to be completed in a reasonable length of time, be portable and should not require expensive accessories or supplies. The objective standardized tests that have been reported in the literature do not meet all of these criteria. Some are limited to the distal extremity function and ignore the shoulder.[3, 4] Others do not specifically concentrate on the upper extremity but include communication disorders, lower extremity deficits and psychosocial problems. The tests that do give a comprehensive picture of the upper extremity require analysis and integration to determine the functional capability.[5, 6] The Functional Test described in this article is intended to be such an assessment. Reliability study of this instrument has been completed and will be reported in a future issue of the American Journal of Occupational Therapy.[7]

THE FUNCTIONAL TEST

The Functional Test consists of seventeen tasks ranging from lifting the involved arm into the lap to using the involved arm to screw in a light bulb. These tasks are arranged in seven levels according to the complexity of motor control required to complete each task. Each level describes the minimum motor control needed to accomplish the tasks it contains. The tasks are arranged within the levels so that each successive item requires a more complex motion. The key motion required and a description of what constitutes successful completion appears with each task. The maximum time allowed for each task is three minutes, but the patient is permitted three attempts at each activity. The test is administered with the patient sitting, preferably in a chair without arms. All items that require manipulation of objects on a table top are performed with patients seated at a standard height table.

Level one: At this level the patient is unable to initiate any voluntary movement of the upper extremity to complete any of the tasks.

Level two: Tasks at this level require beginning voluntary motion of the shoulder and elbow. The first task in this level involves eliciting an associated reaction in the involved extremity by stressing the uninvolved arm. It is the only item in the test that is not voluntarily initiated by the patient, but is therapist induced. The second task at this level requires the patient to place his hand into his lap from a position at his side. The key motion for the "hand into lap" task is a combination of active shoulder and elbow motion. A patient is graded as successful if he places his hand in his lap or on the thigh. If the patient is unable to adequately raise his hand to the level of his lap he is graded as not completing the task, although he makes some attempt.

Level three: Tasks at this level require a mass flexion synergy of at least thirty to sixty degrees of shoulder abduction, sixty to one hundred degrees of elbow flexion, and a minimum of three to five pounds of gross grasp. The simplest task requires the patient to actively move his arm out of the way by abducting his shoulder in a flexion synergy in order to tuck his shirt into the waistband on the involved side. The second task requires a patient to hold a pouch for a specified period of time using gross grasp. The third, and more complex, task requires the combined use of the shoulder and hand motions in order to stabilize a pillow while applying a case.

Level four: Tasks at this level require some elbow extension and one-half to three pounds of lateral pinch as well as the movements already described in the previous levels. The three tasks for this level are to stabilize a jar while opening it, stabilize a package while wrapping it, and wringing excess water from a cloth or rag. The patient is not successful with the jar task, if he braces the jar between his legs rather than stabilize it with his involved arm; or if the patient is unable to grip the jar sufficiently with the uninvolved hand to remove the lid.

Level five: Tasks at this level require the beginning ability to combine components of a strong mass flexion and extension synergies, grasp greater than five pounds and lateral pinch of three pounds, and voluntary release from grasp. The tasks for this level involve holding a lid on a pan while draining liquids, hooking and zipping up a cardigan style garment and assisting the uninvolved extremity in folding a sheet.

Level six: Tasks at this level require isolated control of the shoulder, elbow, and wrist against gravity; full extension of the shoulder, elbow, wrist and fingers; and, greater than five pounds of grasp and three pounds of lateral pinch. The tasks are placing blocks in a box at table height, a box on an overhead shelf, and a coin in a pay telephone coin gauge. The test uses the outdated coin gauges that requires horizontal coin placement because it requires more precise wrist, finger and thumb control.

Level seven: Tasks for the seventh and final level require isolated control of all upper extremity musculature with good coordination and control. The new motion required is isolated manipulation of individual digits and the ability to perform rapid reciprocal motions of the forearm, wrist and hand. Tasks include making a "cat's cradle", screwing a light bulb into a socket, and removing a rubber band from around the palm of the same hand using only finger manipulation.

Grading: The patient is given a plus or a minus for each task. A plus indicates that the patient successfully completes the task within the prescribed three minutes; a minus indicates that he could not complete the activity or exceeded the allowed time. A patient is deemed to be in a given level when he can complete all the tasks it contains. He is not placed into a higher level until he is able to complete *all* the tasks at the next stage. For example, a patient who completes all three tasks in level two would remain a level two patient until he successfully completes the three tasks specified in level three. The test does not attempt to measure all factors necessary to complete these functional tasks, only the motor control components. However, valuable information about perception and cognition can be obtained through observation of the patient's approach to the task and the use of problem solving abilities during performance. The examiner is encouraged to use verbal and visual cues to make up for any deficits the patient may have in perception, vision or cognition.

Instruction manual: To ensure the reliability of the test results, the twenty page manual provides standard instructions for test administration and grading. The manual also contains a list of the materials needed for the test. All the materials can be stored in a box that is 12″ × 6″ × 8″ deep. This makes the Functional Test completely portable and, therefore, practical for use at the patient's bedside, in the treatment clinic, as well as in nursing homes or in the patients' own homes.

RESEARCH NEEDS

The research to be published shows that the Functional Test correlated very highly with objective measures of elbow and wrist joint range of motion, wrist extensor strength, active shoulder flexion and abduction, two-point discrimination and proprioception in the fingers, and spasticity in the elbow, and hand.

Further research is needed to determine if the Functional Test could be used alone as a guide to treatment and obviate numerous assessments currently used by occupational therapists. The key motions that are required for each task as well as the sensory and perceptual requirements need to be validated in order to strengthen the test results. Finally, comparison of the patient's overall functional level in self care and pre-vocational skills to his level on the Functional Test would give the test some predictive value for final treatment outcomes.

SUMMARY

A Functional Test that assesses the use of the hemiparetic upper extremity in purposeful tasks has been described. The implication of its use as an alternative to other commonly used assessment methods has been discussed. The need for further study and refinement has been outlined since this would add to the test's value as an assessment tool for clinical occupational therapists.

Resources

The length of the instruction manual precludes inclusion of its contents totally in this article. Detailed Functional Test instructions and equipment lists are available from: The Professional Staff Association, Rancho Los Amigos Hospital, 7413 Golondrinas Avenue, Downey, California 90242.

REFERENCES

1. Hayes CA, Kassimir J, Parkin J: Sample Forms for Occupational Therapy. Division of Professional Development, American Occupational Therapy Association, Rockvill, MD, 1980.

2. Caldwell CB, Wilson DJ, Braun RM: Evaluation and Treatment of the Upper Extremity in the Hemiplegic Stroke Patient. *J Bone Joint Surg* 63:69-93, 1969.

3. Bell E, Jurek K, Wilson T: Hand Skill Measurements: A Gauge for Treatment. *Am J Occup Ther* 30:80-86, 1976.

4. Jebsen RH, Taylor N, Trieschmann RB, et al: An Objective and Standardized Test of Hand Function. *Arch Phys Med Rehab* 50:311-319, 1969.

5. Bard G, Hirschberg GG, Tolleson GCB: Functional Testing of the Hemiplegic Arm. *Phys Ther* 44:1081-1086, 1964.

6. Kent BE: Sensory Motor Testing: The Upper Limb of Adult Patients with Hemiplegia. *Phys Ther* 45:550-561, 1965.

7. Wilson DJ, Baker LL, Craddock JA: Functional Test for the Hemiparetic Upper Extremity. Submitted to *Am J Occup Ther,* 1983.

Adult Skills Evaluation Survey (ASES) for Persons with Mental Retardation

Jane T. Herrick, BA, OTR
Helen E. Lowe, BS, OTR

ABSTRACT. This paper explains the reasons for developing an assessment tool that would answer the increasingly apparent need for an evaluation instrument to measure developmental levels of performance in programs training adults with mental impairment but little physical disability. The four sections of the assessment are described in terms of content and concepts. The results indicate findings from four years of testing and retesting, providing data useful for appropriate placement in therapy services, for writing measurable goals, for recording progress and for programming tailored to the needs of both individual trainees and groups. The unique contributions of occupational therapists in this field are discussed.

"Mental retardation is not a general phenomenon. Every person labeled retarded has areas of normal capability, developed or undeveloped."[1]

The Adult Skills Evaluation Survey (ASES) was developed by two occupational therapists in a work activity facility training adults with a primary diagnosis of mental retardation. Its purpose was to serve as a guide in program placement and as an aid in measuring the improvement of performance. As well stated by Robert Perske, "The highest dignity and greatest joy in living comes not from trying to be what others are, but from developing into the best persons we can be with the unique strengths and weaknesses we possess."[2]

During the four years it has been in use, ASES has provided data for an interdisciplinary team engaged in planning and carrying out a

---

Jane T. Herrick is a Client Evaluation Specialist at New Opportunity Workshops, Inc., 130 North Fair Oaks Avenue, Pasadena, California 91103. Helen E. Lowe is the Coordinator of Special Projects at New Opportunity Workshops, Inc., 130 North Fair Oaks Avenue, Pasadena, California 91103.

program to promote growth and development in a population of clients with moderate to severe mental dysfunction, but with little overt physical disability.

The problems in dealing with this target group were seen as: incompleteness of case histories, ineffectiveness of traditional interview methods, and lack of a short but comprehensive assessment in the areas of fine motor, perceptual, academic and living skills. Research of available tests showed the majority to be directed toward the child with retardation. Those for adults focused primarily on work skills instead of the whole person.

Assessment of achievement levels in these four areas was seen by the therapists as essential in evaluating current performance and in ascertaining the means to promote growth toward personal, social and work goals. Assessment is vital in discovering the basic skills necessary for purposeful activity and a growth in independence. The data from the survey have been useful as a predictive measure of success for persons whose abilities are such that they are best served at the work activity level.

DESCRIPTION

The assessment consists of four sections which focus on specific performance areas related to the use of small hand muscles, neurological development, academic fundamentals and the practical tasks of everyday living. The scoring is based on a six-point scale from 0 to 5. The lowest score indicates no concept and no ability. The highest score shows performance at or above the top level of the assessment. It has been used with newly admitted clients and as an annual re-test to document gains and losses. The entire test should take no more than two hours to administer. Further data for standardization are being accumulated and the assessment will then be available for publication.

Fine Motor Skills

This section presents six items that represent the type of activities which experience indicates are most predictive of the prevocational expectations of adults with developmental disabilities who are training in work activity programs. One example is bead stringing to assess finger dexterity and bi-manual ability. Another line item is packaging eyelets which evaluates eye-hand coordination and the speed of completing a task. The structured tasks evaluate the functional ability of hands and eyes to perform with skill and ease work which requires finger dexterity, bilaterality, accuracy, speed and strength.

Perceptual Skills

This unit is made up of nine factors that produce a collection of data to evaluate perceptual deficits and assess how much an inefficient sensory system has affected developmentally acquired skills and performance capacities. Matching and collating tasks are included in the first six subtests which are ordered by level of difficulty to quickly pinpoint areas of deficiency and reflect the lack of abilities important to the functioning of auditory and visual perception. Other items give evidence of the awareness of body image and show the degree to which sensory input and motor output have been delayed. Attention deficits are observed by a series of commands requiring listening and responding in a given sequential order.

Academic Skills

The eleven components of this section provide a record of the integration of learning experiences and assess the degree of influence the impairment has exerted on academic achievement. Language and content are appropriate to allow easy scoring of acquired knowledge up to the third grade level and to provide an objective measure of the concepts and splinter skills maintained from previous training. From personal statistics and color identification to the use of numbers, words, time and money, the scores reveal the functional academic skills that are currently useful and those which are minimal or can be improved.

Living Skills

This section surveys six different functions that are essential to managing semi-independence. The items are indicators of dependency and offer guidelines for training towards purposeful activity. Included are several common signs such as traffic lights and restroom identification, also basic self-care items to project the level of competence and independence achieved thus far. Using a telephone and selected hand tools further indicate knowledge of a variety of practical situations encountered in life. Kitchen tasks show the ability to handle everyday household needs.

RESULTS

Mental deficiency causes a serious inability to deal with the environment as a consequence of a brain not performing functions needed to make independent life possible.[3] By using this structured survey to assess dysfunction, specific problems interfering with learning the skills necessary for independent action were discovered and placement in a beneficial program was facilitated.

The data formed the basis for developmental programming with groups of clients most of whom had progressed from school failure to hospitalization, to community placement, to stagnation and were in a sense, frozen in time.[4] The use of the developmental model meant minimal gains could be monumental as a part of survival learning. These gains were an effort to improve the limited behavioral repertoire of persons with mental retardation whose corresponding feelings of helplessness were a limiting factor in their everyday lives.[4]

Results from testing indicated that all of the clients in the work activity center were functionally below a developmental level of eight years in some of the items tested. On the Fine Motor Skills section, 45% of the clients scored at or above the top level of the Survey. In the Perceptual Skills area, 25% of the clients performed at this top level and 20% of the clients were able to successfully complete the Academic Skills and Living Skills sections. Annual re-testing indicates the percentage of improvement of performance in adults with mental retardation is minimal. The greatest progress has occurred in the areas of fine motor and perceptual skills.

The value of ASES as a resource tool in providing information for planning individual short and long term goals has been proven by its usefulness for placement in habilitation groups such as functional academics, sensory motor training and activities of daily living. The production skills tested predicted success in manipulation, reasoning, perception, number and word concepts and work tolerance. During the four years it has been administered, the data from 84 client evaluations and the re-testing of 55 clients have been recorded and have become the basis for graphs depicting the assets and deficits of this group whose cognitive, perceptual and motor deficits indicate a need for continued remediation.

DISCUSSION

The assessment provides data for analyzing and interpreting individual assets and deficiencies. Its length, approximately two hours, is appropriate to the needs of individuals who are functioning at or below a developmental age of eight years, and its format of 77 core items is well adapted to assess the dysfunction that is interfering with learning the skills necessary for productive performance. The nonstressful test setting encourages maximum achievement and behavior to determine those needs which can be most influenced by training. Of equal value is that the assessment allows classification of trainees by ability levels for the purpose of providing services appropriate to their capacities and vital to their potential and quality of life.

Data suggest that more should be done to increase the level and value of the work the retarded do instead of trying to develop bigger and better reinforcement systems for simple, low-paying work.[1] Find out the abilities, capacities and interests of the individual and then help to develop them fully. Every mentally deficient person carries with him a particular combination of abilities, interests and desires.[3] The primary difficulties experienced by the adult disabled are related to the problems of everyday living. The factors causing this are the inherent limitations in dealing with concepts and language, immature habits, the age factor and inadequate living environments. Overall, observations from testing outcomes indicate these interesting and thought-provoking generalities: clients possess the ability to perform simple tasks with their hands in spite of poor ocular control, have good matching skills, poor reasoning, difficulty in following verbal directions, little ability to read, write, count, compute, make change and tell time.

Occupational therapists, with their orientation toward persons with developmentally disabling conditions and impaired performance, are well equipped to use an assessment of this kind. Therapists feel a responsibility to identify needs, analyze problems and implement goals essential for the optimum level of function. The compactness of this tool decreases documentation time and permits the examiner to readily evaluate existing function, interpret results and observe the degree of adaptation employed by the subject. Mae D. Hightower-Vandamm has written that the occupational therapist has a role in the evaluation of physically and mentally handicapped clients through the provision of a functional evaluation and a sensorimotor evaluation where indicated and through the management of a sustaining evaluation program.[5] The assessment becomes a living laboratory as the findings permit enough diversity of information to be continually useful for charting comparisons when new program ideas surface. Individual scores are considered as important as the whole, all the while using caution not to fragment the client, but dealing simultaneously with all the factors that disrupt his performance and give attention to his needs as a total person.

Besides investigating prevocational skills, the assessment has a strong emphasis on habilitation concepts. Overlooking these would cause a lack of awareness of the basic developmental problems and thereby lead to further disability or a failure to recognize the barriers that limit cognitive and social roles. Because of the tendency of the performer to perceive in other ways than he was expected to perceive, he distorted what he saw, heard, drew, tasted and smelled. He perceived something, but not what was expected.[6] This results in the inability to follow verbal directions, to process visual information and to gain knowledge from the environment for the purposes of learning.

CONCLUSION

The service provided by this assessment is worthwhile to the agency and beneficial to the recipient. Promoting growth and determining progress are legitimate occupational therapy objectives in community based training programs. For persons with mental retardation intellectual ability in adulthood may have reached a point of little or no advancement. Nonetheless, motivating people to learn through purposeful occupational therapy to perform essential tasks and find a place in productive living is the challenging and most rewarding role of the occupational therapist.

REFERENCES

1. Gold M: *Try Another Way,* Austin, Tx: Mark Gold & Associates Inc., 1980.
2. Perske R: *Hope for the Families,* Nashville, TN: Abingdon Press, 1981.
3. Isaacson R: *Meeting the Needs of the Retarded,* Niles, Il: Argus Communications, 1977.

4. Kielhofner G: The Temporal Dimension of the Lives of Retarded Adults: A Problem of Interaction and Intervention: *Am. J. Occup. Ther.* 33:161-169, 1979.

5. Vandamm M: The Role of Occupational Therapy in Vocational Evaluation, Part 2: *Am. J. Occup. Ther.* 35:631-633.

6. Barsch R: *Achieving Perceptual Motor Efficiency* (Vol. 1), Seattle, Wa: Special Child Publications, 1963.

A Description of an Occupational Therapy Program for Students with Disabilities Who Attend a Community College

Sandra Burnett-Beaulieu, MA, OTR

ABSTRACT. An occupational therapy program for community college students who are disabled is described. The non-traditional program utilizes physical and psycho-social assessments to assist in treatment planning. Student role fulfillment is the central goal of treatment. The organizational context, the population served, and the assessment and therapy process are discussed. The description is designed to aid those who seek to develop community-based, treatment programs.

The assessment procedures and the types of information needed to establish effective treatment programs are shaped by the practice setting. Occupational therapists have always served individuals with disabilities. The trend for such individuals to be included in mainstream life (e.g., school, work, recreation) expands the role of occupational therapy into settings other than medical facilities. The following is an account of the ways a novel practice setting, a community college, has shaped a therapy process.

At Santa Monica College (SMC) a non-traditional occupational

Sandra Burnett-Beaulieu is currently the Registered Occupational Therapist for the Disabled Students' Center at Santa Monica College, Santa Monica, California and Clinical Assistant Professor, Occupational Therapy Department at the University of Southern California, Los Angeles, California.

The author and the program are deeply indebted to the vision and encouragement of Elizabeth J. Yerxa, EdD, OTR and Judith Schwartz, PhD.

therapy program for community college students who are disabled was initiated in 1978.* First, a descriptive survey was conducted in cooperation with several public and private agencies serving disabled individuals. The survey determined the self-perceived needs of physically disabled persons. This served as a preliminary step in designing for occupational therapy intervention at the community college. Significant differences in the confidence to perform cognitive/problem-solving, social/recreational, school/vocational, home and community mobility skills were found when the disabled persons were compared with nondisabled, student counterparts.[1]

This paper is a description of the intervention program which has evolved during the last five years. A trend toward community health care by occupational therapists, contrasted with hospital based practice, was highlighted by Cromwell and Keilhofner.[2] The objective of this program description is to aid those who seek to establish similar community-based programs.

ORGANIZATIONAL CONTEXT

Since the mid-1970's all California community colleges have received state funding to provide specialized services for students who are disabled. Santa Monica Community College District funds are also contributed to sustain the program. The Handicapped Student Programs and Services (HSP&S) are primarily directed by counselors and educators who are mandated to facilitate the "mainstreaming" of disabled students into academic and vocational courses of instruction and into general campus programs. The most common methods used by colleges to achieve that directive are counseling, tutoring, providing special equipment and parking privileges, designing barrier-free environments, and instruction of pre-college, preparatory courses designed specifically for students who are disabled. In addition, almost all the community colleges offer adaptive physical education courses for disabled students. Many colleges conduct special assessment and support services for students with learning disabilities.

---

*The project was initiated under a United States Department of Health Education and Welfare (HEW), Rehabilitation Services Administration training grant awarded to the University of Southern California Occupational Therapy Department.

POPULATION SERVED

The nomenclature itself used to identify those who are served by the occupational therapy program reflects a shift in approach. *Students* who attend the college and who are disabled, not patients or clients, are eligible for occupational therapy services. The population is defined by role identification, namely, being a student, and by a second criteria, namely, those having some type of medically or educationally recognized disability. Thus, role dysfunction and activities which promote role fulfillment are the central themes of occupational assessment and intervention practices rather than treatment based solely upon medical etiology and pathology.[3]

The students who are served by the program usually have a severe physical disability, such as multiple sclerosis, cerebral palsy, traumatic head injury, cerebral vascular accident, or spinal cord injury. Students with learning disabilities also are provided some services. The students served range in age from 18 years to retirement years. Most are young adults seeking to develop skills which will lead to employment, independence from their nuclear families, and a satisfying social life. Intervention is designed in accordance with the self-stated goals of the student. The approach, for example, will differ for a 19 year old youth who has had a head injury, is an art major, and is aspiring to become an architect as opposed to a 65 year old person with residuals from a cerebral vascular accident who is taking an art class for recreation. Thus the developmental stages and the self-stated goals of the students are crucial ingredients for program planning.

THERAPY PROCESS

Identification

Approximately 500 students voluntarily seek support services from the HSP&S office at SMC each year. Most of the students are interviewed and counseled by an academic counselor who is a specialist with disabled students. One of the first tasks undertaken when occupational therapy services were new in the setting was to clarify for the counselors the types of services the occupational therapist could offer so that the counselor could refer students appropriately. Initially a checklist of skills which might be problems for students was given to the counselor. Using that checklist during the initial interview, the counselor directs questions which reveal whether or not a student should be referred to occupational therapy. The initial counselor checklist items were drawn from the needs survey questionnaire.[1]

The counselor then sends a referral slip to the occupational therapist mentioning both initial checklist problems, specific classroom situations which may present problems (e.g., wheelchair user enrolled in data processing) and a request for an evaluation by the therapist. The occupational therapist then contacts the student. It is important to note that services are non-prescriptive. The student is assisted by the counselor in identifying his problems but then must take the step of availing himself of help. The assessment process, in a community setting such as this, begins with the individual's ability to want assistance with problem areas. Neither further assessment nor treatment can proceed without that initial desire by the individual. The college program encourages the student to keep the responsibility for seeking assistance both because it is congruent with an adult life stage and it is therapeutically supportive of his sense of efficacy.[4]

Initial Assessment

An individual assessment of each student referred is conducted by a Registered Occupational Therapist. The starting point for all assessments is consideration of 1) the student's self-stated goals for attending the college and 2) a self-report of current (or anticipated) problems he has performing skills required for life roles, e.g., student, homemaker, roommate, worker. Assessment is carried out in four major areas: physical, emotional, cognitive function and occupational history.[5] A self-report questionnaire, the Yerxa et. al., Satisfaction with Performance Scaled Questionnaire,[6] developed specifically for use with college students who are disabled, is used both as a problem identification tool and as a pre-test measure. Information from other professionals providing services for the student is obtained when available. (In a community setting it is particularly important to know which other professionals are providing counseling, therapy, etc., to the student so that a coordinated "team" approach can occur). Other assessments are used when appropriate. For example, a Time Log[7] may be required when the student has problems with time management; an Interest Checklist[8] may be administered if avenues for social contact, the development of a hobby, or a craft activity for treatment are desired or needed; Allen's Cognitive Levels assessment[9] has been used with learning disabled students to identify the appropriate methods of instruction in independent living skills.

The data from the initial assessment are used by the therapist to formulate a treatment plan. Treatment goals and their expected dates of completion are recorded. Referral to other professionals both at the college (e.g., psychologist for symptoms of depression) and outside the college (e.g., rehabilitation center occupational therapy for a splinting evaluation) may be part of the plan.

Treatment Approaches

Several approaches are employed by the occupational therapist to pursue treatment goals. Individual sessions are set up to instruct students in skills, such as the use of equipment, handwriting and typing, or energy conservation. Workshops for small groups of students are conducted (for four to ten sessions) to cover topics such as money management and leisure interest exploration. Elective, college credit semester courses are also taught. These include Basic Food Preparation and Independent Living Skills (ILS). (The instructional materials used for the ILS course have been produced in a manual.[6])**

The occupational therapy program also provides consultation to the instructor in the Adaptive Physical Education course. The occupational therapist's knowledge of precautions associated with various diagnoses is valuable for this procedure. Together with the instructor and students, individualized goals for participation in the course are established in a contractual format. The student must have authorization to enroll in the course by a physician. All classroom aides in adaptive P.E. classes receive training sessions from the occupational therapists. Such topics as basic exercise principles, transfer techniques and attitudes towards disability are covered in those sessions.

Another role the occupational therapist serves in this setting is to contact the college faculty of both the vocational and academic pro-

**The project which developed the manual was funded by a grant from the California State Chancellor's Office, Fund for Improvement of Instruction.

grams each year to encourage the discussion of concerns they are having about individual students who are disabled. The confidentiality of the student's disability is maintained in those discussions by focusing on specific class-related difficulties and methods which might be used to improve performance. The importance of including both the instructor and the student in the problem-solving process is a basic principle that is stressed.

Review and Coordination

There are two ways in which the occupational therapy program is assessed for its effectiveness and its value as part of the educational service delivery system. The primary function of the college is to provide education and vocational training. Thus all support services, all non-academic programs, are evaluated by whether they are assisting students and faculty in fulfilling *educational* goals. At the college during the past five years there has been a continuous review of this program by faculty and administrators, judging its value for the entire college community. It has been found that both the faculty member who is able to depend upon help with a problem student and the student who must develop skills necessary to function independently as a college student have been served effectively. Each has reduced fears and increased competence in the tasks required in their interaction with one another.

A second arena for program review has been within the larger community of agencies and professionals who serve those students with disabilities. In many instances the occupational therapy program has been a bridge between medical rehabilitation and life in the mainstream. Dialogues between medical rehabilitation service providers and the college support staff about the ways all can serve the students' needs has increased since initiation of the occupational program. Further, the occupational therapist can act as a catalyst in helping students move from the discharge recommendations and out-patient follow-up of his medical rehabilitation providers to the demands of college life. This function has been achieved through interdisciplinary case conferences about particular students and information sharing sessions between staffs during which their respective service functions are discussed. In this way gaps in service for assisting students to acquire requisite skills for college life can be identified and the transition between medical support and college demands can be bridged. Thus the value of the occupational therapy program is made visible to the community service providers and is assessed by them as well as by the college community.

CONCLUSION

The program described is an example of one way in which the occupational therapist's skills and knowledge base can be utilized in a non-traditional setting. Role dysfunction and activities which promote role fulfillment are central themes of occupational therapy assessment and treatment practices rather than treatment based solely upon medical etiology and pathology. The description is *not* a prescription for how a program at a community college must be conducted. Rather it is hoped that it will serve as an example of some of the ways in which a community-based treatment program can be integrated into the ecology of a non-traditional setting.

REFERENCES

1. Burnett SE, Yerxa EJ: Community-based and college-based needs assessment of physically disabled persons, *Am J Occ Therapy* 34:201-207, 1980.
2. Cromwell FS, Kielhofner GW: An educational strategy for occupational therapy community service, *Am J Occ Therapy* 30:629-633, 1976.
3. Black MM: The occupational career . . ., *Am J Occ Therapy* 30:225-228, 1976.
4. Burke JP: A clinical perspective on motivation: Pawn versus origin, *Am J Occ Therapy* 31:254-258, 1977.
5. Moorehead L: The occupational history, *Am J Occ Therapy* 23:329-332, 1969.
6. Burnett SE: *Seven Modules for Independent Living Skills Instruction for Physically Disabled College Students,* Santa Monica, CA: Disabled Students' Center, Santa Monica College, July, 1982.
7. Larrington G: *An Exploratory Study of the Temporal Aspects of Adaptive Functioning,* University of Southern California, Occupational Therapy Department, Master's Thesis, 1970.
8. Matsutsuyu, JS: Interest Checklist: *Am J Occ Therapy* 23:323-328, 1969.
9. Allen CK: Interdependence through activity: The practice of occupational therapy (psychiatry), *Am J Occ Therapy* 36:731-739, 1982.

Physiological Monitoring: Assessment of Energy Cost

Kathleen C. Shanfield, MA, OTR

ABSTRACT. Many patients with physical disabilities are limited by poor endurance. This could be due to the level of deconditioning, the disease or injury, and/or the demands of the activities they must perform. Occupational therapists historically have been involved in the study of energy cost of activities and have used such concepts in prescribing activity and teaching energy conservation. The purpose of this paper is to (1) review briefly the study of energy cost and its significance to occupational therapy practice and (2) to describe the Physiological Monitored Evaluation (PME). The PME can be used to assess the demands of activities on patients by measuring the heart rate, blood pressure, and symptomatic responses to activities. This procedure can be used to obtain baseline measurements to compare and document progress, set safe guidelines for activity so that the patient may increase endurance without becoming "overstressed", and collect data for research.

How can the demands of activity on the patient be determined? What tools are available to assess changes in the patient's work tolerance? How can occupational therapists assess whether a treatment program is safe yet adequate to increase endurance? These are common questions asked by therapists engaged in intervention programs with patients limited by poor endurance. Because the occupational therapist uses activities of all kinds as treatment, it is important to know their energy costs in order to select and use activities in a safe yet effective manner. Thus the Physiological Monitored Evaluation (PME) was developed as an assessment strategy which can be applied in many treatment settings.

The purpose of this paper is to (1) briefly review the study of energy cost and its significance to occupational therapy practice, and (2) describe the Physiological Monitored Evaluation (PME) as a

Kathleen C. Shanfield, OTR, holds an MA in Exercise Physiology, and is currently practicing at Daniel Freeman Hospital in Inglewood, CA.

tool that therapists can use to assess the stress of activities on any patient.

THE STUDY OF ENERGY COST

"Cost" of work is measured in terms of energy used. Energy can be measured and described by (1) determining units of heat production or calories used, (2) ascertaining the volume of O_2 consumed (VO_2), or Metabolic Equivalents (METS) and/or (3) monitoring physiological variables such as heart rate (HR) and blood pressure (BP) with activity.

Energy cost studies date back to the early 1900's, yet it was not until the 1950's that these data were applied to rehabilitation. Due to the expensive equipment and trained personnel required to collect the data, these studies were limited in scope. Subjects were usually young and healthy, and population samples were small. Many investigators commented on the wide variability in data among subjects performing the same activity.[1] Nevertheless, tables of activities and their estimated energy cost in terms of calories used, the VO_2, or METS were devised.[2]

Occupational therapists commonly have used these tables as guidelines in prescribing activity programs and/or teaching energy conservation. However, the data do not account for individual differences due to age, sex, weight, or physical condition.[3] Neither do they consider factors inherent in an activity that can increase energy cost by causing the heart rate (HR) and blood pressure (BP) to rise faster than otherwise expected. These factors include: using the arms (especially overhead), isometric contractions, level of skill and pace, holding the breath or Valsalva, emotional stress, and environmental conditions such as heat and cold.[4-7] Most activities of daily living (ADL) will include one or more of these factors. Studies with the disabled population show that additional factors such as pain, joint limitations, spasticity, muscle weakness or loss, and excessive use of the arms will increase the energy used during ambulation.[8, 9] No studies to date have measured the energy cost of self-care or other daily living activities performed by patients.

PHYSIOLOGICAL MONITORED EVALUATION

Occupational therapists can assess energy cost and demands that activities make or put on patients by the Physiological Monitored Evaluation (PME). PME is a method of evaluating the HR, BP, and symptomatic responses to activity. This procedure can be used to (1) obtain baseline measurements with which to compare or document progress, (2) set safe guidelines for activity so that the patient may increase endurance without being "overstressed," and (3) collect data for research. This tool is commonly used with cardiac patients; however, the concept and procedure is appropriate for any patient with poor endurance, for example, those with pulmonary disease, stroke, the debilitating problems of aging and spinal injury.

The clinical parameters assessed are the HR, BP, and symptoms such as shortness of breath (SOB), pain, angina, or fatigue. Electrocardiographic (EKG) monitoring with telemetry can also be valuable because it can detect arrhythmias, ischemia, and yield an accurate HR during activity.[10]

Heart Rate and Blood Pressure

The HR is probably the best tool available to measure energy cost and stress on the patient.[11] HR can be influenced by medications, food, caffeine, cigarettes, and heat. Therefore, it is used ideally as a measure of function in conjunction with the BP. The HR can be obtained by taking the pulse, using EKG telemetry, or with commercially available pulse meters.

To obtain an accurate pulse, the therapist should be familiar with where the radial or carotid pulse can be felt immediately after activity. Then one counts the beats for ten seconds, starting the count at zero, multiplies this number by six to obtain the number of beats per minute (bpm's). Obtaining the pulse and BP's immediately after activity requires practice and concentration. Ideally one therapist and an assistant perform the PME, one taking BP's and the other checking HR. If only one therapist is available, the HR should be taken first, followed immediately by a BP.

Symptoms

Correlating symptoms with HR and BP gives an added functional dimension to physical capacity. Reporting symptoms can be very subjective; however, scales can be devised to quantify responses. Two scales which have been found to be helpful are the Shortness of Breath (SOB) Index,[12] and Borg's Rate of Perceived Exertion (RPE) Scale.[13]

The SOB Index (Figure 1) was devised by the Cardio-Pulmonary Team at Rancho Los Amigos Hospital to quantify dyspnea. The pa-

Figure 1: Shortness of Breath Index (15 count)

Level 1	Urgency
Level 2	Needs one breath
Level 3	Needs two or more
Level 4	Can't talk

tient is asked to count to fifteen in one breath immediately after activity. If the patient rushes through the count in one breath, this is Level 1. If the patient takes one breath during the count, Level 2, two breaths, Level 3, and inability to talk is Level 4. Borg's RPE Scale makes possible the quantification of fatigue (Figure 2). The patient is shown the scale after performing activity and asked to rate subjectively how much effort the activity demanded. RPE Levels increase linearly with the workload and correlation with HR is high ($r = .80—.90$, $p < .05$).[13] Many investigators have confirmed the HR/RPE relationship and this scale is widely used by exercise physiologists. Both of these scales also can be used by the patient as pacing tools.

Activity Choice

Activities to be monitored are determined by the patient's functional abilities and goals, as well as factors inherent in the tasks that may increase energy cost. Functional abilities and goals can be obtained by (1) the medical chart review, (2) the occupational therapy interview and (3) observation. "Red flags" that indicate possible problems with endurance and/or fatigue are: a history of cardiovascular or pulmonary problems, muscle loss or atrophy, depression, malnutrition, inactivity for more than two weeks, pain and/or a high resting pulse. A survey of daily activities and interests should include specific questions regarding symptoms during performance of those activities, i.e., fatigue, SOB, dizziness, pain, etc. Observation of the patients' mobility, sitting tolerance, affect, and SOB with talking can give clues to the patients' level of endurance.

For the patient with very low endurance, and/or cardiac problems, the initial monitoring of basic self-care tasks will provide a good indication of physiologic responses to any light activity. If no problems are detected, more activities can be added to the program, using the PME for each new activity.

For patients with specific activity/fatigue problems, the PME can be used to assess those specific activities. The following is a list of specific activities that patients commonly find fatiguing and thus are commonly assessed by the PME.

Figure 2: Borg's Rating of Perceived Exertion (RPE) Scale

6	
7	Very very light
8	
9	Very light
10	
11	Fairly light
12	
13	Somewhat hard
14	
15	Hard
16	
17	Very hard
18	
19	Very very hard
20	

—Self Care: dressing—upper and lower extremities, hygiene and grooming, bathing, transfers, Valsalva.
—Home Maintenance: reaching and placing objects into cabinets—upper and lower, sweeping, vacuuming, washing dishes, carrying trash, laundry, lawn mowing, gardening.
—Vocational: hammering, sawing, pipe fitting, car repair, lifting, pushing/pulling specific objects/weights.
—Recreational: dancing—slow and fast, fishing—casting and reeling, wood-working and other crafts, golf, bowling.

Physiologic and symptomatic responses are recorded (1) after activity is completed, or (2) at five minute work intervals until task is completed and/or (3) when patient becomes symptomatic. The patient is encouraged to work at his normal pace. The initial PME should include responses to tasks performed without assistance or modifications. A baseline is then established and problem areas can be identified. The PME should be discontinued if (1) the HR exceeds 180 bpm and/or (2) the BP exceeds 220/110 or drops below 90/60, and/or (3) symptoms become uncomfortable.[14]

Guidelines

These general guidelines can be followed for a safe activity program based on the initial PME.

1. Rest for one minute or until responses decrease if the HR increases more than thirty bpm's, and/or the systolic BP increases more than twenty mmHg, and/or the diastolic BP increases more than ten mmHg from the resting values.
2. Post-activity responses should return to resting level within five minutes. If they do not, the demands are probably too great and modifications should be made.[14] Patients with unstable cardiac conditions should follow specific guidelines set by the physician.

CASE EXAMPLE

A.J. is a 70-year-old male three weeks post right CVA with mild residual left hemiparesis. Review of the medical chart revealed the following problems that may indicate poor endurance:

1. Peripheral vascular disease
2. History of hypertension
3. Chronic bronchitis

The initial occupational therapy interview revealed that A.J. is retired and lives with his wife. He was previously independent in all daily living activities and enjoys woodworking, fishing and gardening. Fatigue and SOB have limited these activities for the past year, however. A.J. is presently independent in his basic self-care and his goals are to return to his previous activities in his home and in the community. Observation of self-care tasks indicated that due to the energy and time required to do them he appeared very fatigued.

A treatment program to increase left upper extremity strength and coordination, and to increase overall endurance was planned. A PME during woodworking tasks was performed to establish a baseline of physiologic responses and to determine guidelines for activity (see Figure 3).

The following guidelines were established for the first week:

1. a one minute break every five minutes of activity during the treatment session
2. symptoms not to exceed Level 15 RPE/2 SOB
3. HR and BP should be recorded before and after each treatment session.

Interim PME's were performed at the end of each week and new guidelines set, based on A.J.'s responses. PME's were also used to assess responses during showering, slow dancing with his wife, and with his home exercise program. A.J. was also instructed in body mechanics, pacing techniques, and pulse monitoring.

The discharge PME (see Figure 4) indicated improvement in all physiologic and symptomatic responses, as well as overall endurance.

Improvements or gains in responses may be due to: (1) an increase in physical condition, (2) modifications in doing the activity, that is, better body mechanics, etc. and/or (3) more confidence and familiarity with the tasks. It is important to document evidence of these factors since they reflect the effectiveness of occupational therapy intervention.

Figure 3

Initial PME 1-5-83

Activity		HR	BP	Symptoms	Summary
sitting		90	130/80		Purpose of PME was to establish baseline responses to arm work performed while standing. All HR's and BP's were higher than expected and he fatigued easily. Work tolerance is 5-10 minutes. Patient appears to be deconditioned and uses poor body mechanics and pacing skills.
standing		95	120/75		
sanding	5 min	120	135/90	10 RPE 1 SOB	
painting	5 min	130	150/95	15 RPE 2 SOB	
rest	1 min	105	140/90	1 SOB	
rest	5 min	100	135/90	"tired"	

Discharge PME 2-7-83

Activity		HR	BP	Symptoms	Summary
Sitting	5 min	80	120/75		Patient demonstrates improvement in HR, BP and symptomatic responses, as well as in overall endurance. He is able to work for one hour before requiring a rest, and utilizes good body mechanics and pacing skills.
Standing		85	115/75		
Sanding	5 min	90	130/80	8 RPE 0 SOB	
Sanding	30 min	100	135/85	10 RPE 0 SOB	
Painting	5 min	100	135/85	10 RPE 0 SOB	
Painting	30 min	105	140/85	13 RPE 1 SOB	
Rest	1 min	85	120/75		
Rest	5 min	80	120/75		

Figure 4

DIAGNOSIS

Diagnosis can influence the HR and BP responses to activity. The patient with a stroke may demonstrate high BP responses and the HR may be difficult to determine due to atrial arrhythmias. The patient with chronic obstructive pulmonary disease (COPD) usually shows high HR responses due to the types of medications he takes as well as his level of deconditioning. The spinal injured quadriplegic will show little or no increase in HR due to the decreased autonomic drive.[15] The patient with diabetes and the elderly may also show high BP responses. Any questions regarding abnormal physiological responses should be discussed with the physician so as to set appropriate guidelines.

In summary, this paper has provided a brief review of energy cost studies, and has described the Physiological Monitored Evaluation (PME) as a tool that occupational therapists can use to assess the demands of activities on any patient. The PME could also be used as a research tool to establish typical HR, BP and symptomatic responses to activities performed by patients with different diagnoses. Guidelines for safe activity are often difficult to set due to the lack of data concerning energy cost of activities of daily living. Knowing the demands of tasks on patients can help occupational therapists set realistic treatment goals and, by increasing endurance, one less obstacle to challenge the patients' abilities is removed.

REFERENCES

1. Durnin JVGA, Namyslwoski L: Individual variations in the energy expenditure of standardized activities. J Physiol 143:537-578, 1958.

2. Trombly CA, Scott AD: "Cardiac Rehabilitation" in Occupational Therapy for Physical Dysfunction. Baltimore, MD: Williams and Wilkins, 1977.

3. Passmore R, Durnin JVGA: Human energy expenditure. Physiol Rev 35:801-839, 1955.

4. Henry V: Individual differences in O_2 metabolism of work at two speeds. Res Quart 22:324-333, 1961.

5. Brouha L, Smith PE: Physiological reactions of men and women during muscular activity in various environments. JAP 16:133-140, 1961.

6. Weaver EK: Factors affecting energy expended in home-making tasks. J Am Diet Assoc 39:205, 1961.

7. Ogden LD: Guidelines for Analysis and Testing of ADL with Cardiac Patients. Downey, CA: Cardiac Rehabilitation Inc., 1980.

8. Gordon EE: Energy costs in health and disease. Arch Int Med 101:702-713, 1958.

9. Gilbert D: Energy expenditure for the disabled home-maker: Review of studies. Am J Occup Ther 19:321-327, 1965.

10. Ogden LD: Procedure Guidelines for Monitored Self-Care Evaluation. Downey, CA: Cardiac Rehabilitation, Inc., 1980.

11. Malhotra MS: Pulse count as a measure of energy expenditure. JAP 18:994-996, 1963.

12. Shortness of Breath Index. Physical Therapy Staff, Rancho Los Amigos Hospital, Downey, CA, 1979.

13. Borg GA: Perceived exertion: A note on "history" and methods. Med Sci Sports Sci 5:90-93, 1973.

14. Guidelines for Monitoring of ADL. Occupational Therapy Department Cardiac Service, Rancho Los Amigos Hospital, Downey, CA, 1976.

15. Gass GC, Camp EM: Effects of physical training on high level spinal lesion patients. Scan J Rehabil Med 12, 1980.

Cardiac Work Tolerance Screening: A Case Study

Norma L. Beauchamp, MS, OTR
Cynthia Creighton, MA, OTR
Lori Clark Summers, OTR

ABSTRACT. The transition from inpatient to worker is often a difficult one for the individual recovering from an acute coronary event. While all activities are directed and closely monitored in the hospital, medical recommendations to the convalescent may be as general as, "do anything you want, within your limitations" or "take it easy". By translating such advice into realistic guidelines for performing work tasks, the occupational therapist may reduce a client's uncertainty and encourage him to maintain a healthfully productive life.

This paper describes the assessment procedure used in a community hospital occupational therapy department with a client recovering from an acute myocardial infarction. Methods of job analysis, work simulation and cardiac monitoring which were applied in the assessment are discussed. The use of assessment results to assist the client in returning to his job as an elevator mechanic is explained.

Since the 1960's[1] occupational therapists have been involved in the assessment of the cardiac patient for return to daily life activities. Methods of measuring and regulating the cardiovascular

---

Norma Beauchamp is Assistant Professor of Occupational Therapy at Eastern Michigan University, Ypsilanti, Michigan 48197. Cynthia Creighton is Assistant Professor of Occupational Therapy at Eastern Michigan University, Ypsilanti. Lori Summers is Staff Therapist, Occupational Therapy Section, St. Joseph Mercy Hospital, Ann Arbor, Michigan 48106.

This paper is a modification of a presentation made by the authors at the First Annual Work Capacity Evaluation Conference in St. Louis, Missouri, July 16, 1983.

demands of activity have become increasingly sophisticated. Dempster-Ogden states that functional assessment using modern equipment and research data in exercise physiology is being implemented in several cardiac rehabilitation programs throughout the country.[2] An especially promising method of performing such assessment is the Monitored Task Evaluation developed by the occupational therapy and physical therapy departments of Rancho Los Amigos Hospital in Downey, California. Monitored Task Evaluations have been used to measure cardiac stress during participation in self-care and homemaking tasks.[3] Recently, the Monitored Task Evaluation has been recommended as a major component of the work tolerance screening for cardiac patients returning to the job market. As defined by Matheson, work tolerance screening is "an intensive evaluation of an individual's ability to sustain work performance."[4, p.1] The primary demands of an employment situation are simulated in a controlled environment in which the client demonstrates his response to work as he performs the simulated tasks.

This paper describes the work tolerance screening developed by occupational therapists for one client in the cardiac rehabilitation program of a 558 bed acute care hospital.

CASE STUDY

W. F. is a 52 year old male who suffered a moderate inferior myocardial infarction. He had an uncomplicated hospital course except for an episode of renal insufficiency. The patient was followed by an occupational therapist at the community hospital through a traditional cardiac inpatient and home convalescence program for two and one-half months. He was monitored during this time period performing activity to 5 METs[5] without significant electrocardiographic and hemodynamic changes and without signs or symptoms of intolerance. This is an adequate MET level for performance of most self-care, sedentary leisure, and vocational tasks. Following the home convalescence program, W. F. was given a graded exercise test in which he achieved 11 METs.

During his convalescence, the patient expressed concerns regarding his return to work. He had been employed as an elevator mechanic in a large state university before hospitalization and his employer favored his resuming that position. It was not clear, however, whether or not the required job tasks would be within W. F.'s safe activity level. In order to assess and predict the client's cardiovascular response to performance of critical tasks in his job, a work tolerance screening in occupational therapy seemed appropriate. This provided objective recommendations about his return to work.

Work Tolerance Screening

In order to develop an accurate job simulation for W. F., it was necessary to gather specific information about the work of an elevator mechanic. A variety of methods of data collection was used including an interview with the client and reference to the *Dictionary of Occupational Titles.*[6] An on-site observation was arranged in the elevator repair shop of a local university. During that one hour period an elevator mechanic and his supervisor explained and demonstrated the primary job tasks involved. The occupational therapist recorded the information presented and photographed key tasks and equipment at the job site (Figure 1). Special attention was given to aspects of the job which placed increased demands on the cardiovascular system, e.g., mobility, working against resistance, and extended use of upper extremities at or above shoulder level. The final step in gathering data about the occupation was to confer with the client regarding details, such as the amount of weight lifted, the duration of activities, etc. A questionnaire was developed to record this information (Figure 2).

An analysis of the data collected led to the development of a work tolerance screening for this client which involved simulation of two critical job requirements: stair climbing and electrical wiring at high and low levels. All other routine aspects of elevator repair appeared to be within W. F.'s safe activity level as demonstrated during his home convalescence program and graded exercise test. Five months after his discharge from the hospital, the occupational therapist arranged a job simulation for the patient. Three outpatient clinic visits were scheduled. A modified V-5 chest lead telemetry system (portable ECG monitor) and arm blood pressure cuff were attached to the client to record heart rate, blood pressure and ECG findings at regular intervals. The first job task simulated was wiring at an electrical board. According to the American College of Sports Medicine,[7] wiring is moderate work requiring only 2.5 to 5.5 METs. MET requirements vary with changes in body position and duration of activ-

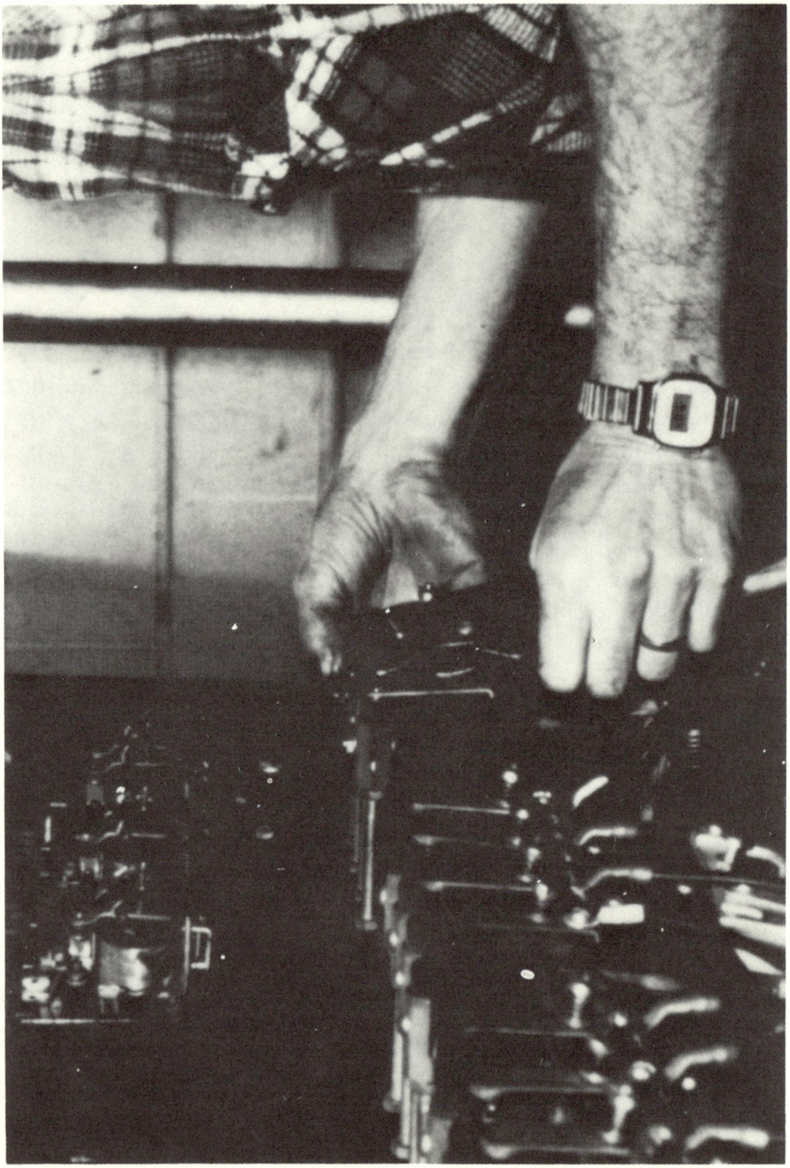

FIGURE 1.

WORK TOLERANCE SCREENING SELF-REPORT

CARDIAC

Name: W. F.

Physician: -

Title of Job: Elevator Mechanic (Group Leader)

Description of Job: Service 3-6 elevators per day on University campus. Load truck and drive it to reach problem area. Climb stairs. "Troubleshoot" at electrical board and in elevator cars, perform routine maintenance and repair of electrical and mechanical parts, act as consultant and leader to less experienced mechanics.

Walking Required: Walk from parked truck to elevator in building, some walking to and from truck and inside buildings.

Frequency: Usually once per elevator (3-6 times per day).

Distance: Up to one block from parking area.

Type of Terrain: Grass, sidewalk, often hilly.

Climbing Stairs/Ladders Required: Climb stairs and some ladders to reach parts.

Frequency: At least once per elevator, may return for additional equipment.

Number of Levels: 2-10 flights per elevator.

Number of Steps: Varies.

Pushing/Pulling Required (include only activity which is maintained for more than 60 seconds): Push and pull loaded safety cart to and from elevator, with partner - infrequently.

Body Position: Standing

Weight of Object: 1,000 lbs.

Lifting/Carrying Required (include only activity which is maintained for more than 60 seconds): Carry tool belt, 2-way radio, light parts.

Distance: Up to 1 block from parking area, up stairs.

Weight of Object: Belt and radio total 15 lbs., parts under 50 lbs.

Levels Lifted To/From: Floor to and from trunk height.

Working with Hands Above Shoulder Level (include only activity which is maintained for more than 60 seconds): Working at higher levels of electrical board.

Duration: Periods of 1/2 hour to 2 hours.

Is the Working Environment Unusually Hot or Cold? Both

Explain: involves walking to buildings in winter, working in unheated parking structures. Old buildings, elevator cars and penthouses may reach 100^{0} or more in summer.

What Are the Most Stressful or Demanding Aspects of the Job?

Physical Stressors: Climbing and occasional lifting and pulling of heavy equipment.

Emotional Stressors: Managing people trapped in elevators, worries about fire in buildings, people who do not understand or respect equipment.

Environmental Stressors: Heat and cold.

FIGURE 2.

ity, however, and it was felt that the more demanding aspects of this task should be observed. To simulate wiring, available tools and materials were used. A Bennett Hand Tool Dexterity test board was placed six inches from the floor on the shelf of a cabinet.[8] W. F. removed and replaced the bolts with hand tools. He wore a two-pound weight attached to his belt to simulate the walkie-talkie that elevator mechanics carry while working. No significant changes in ECG, blood pressure or heart rate were noted in six minutes, so the Test was placed on another shelf at the client's shoulder level (Figure 3). Again, W. F. tolerated the activity well.

The second job function simulated was stair climbing, since in his work, W. F. was required to climb as many as ten flights of stairs at a time, several times each day. A set of training stairs was used for the simulation. The client was asked to demonstrate the pace which was typical for him on the job, wearing his own tool belt and the two-pound weight. The demonstration indicated that W. F. typically climbed at an energy cost of approximately 12 METs (65 steps per minute on an eight inch rise, carrying 15 pounds), which exceeded the 11 METs that he had achieved previously on his graded exercise test. It was decided that the simulation could be safely continued, because there had been no symptoms of cardiac stress other than fatigue when the exercise test was discontinued. W. F. was monitored carefully as he climbed (Figure 4). After three minutes, he began to experience shortness of breath and fatigue. The ECG showed normal sinus rhythm with rare premature ventricular contractions and nonspecific T-wave changes. The client was also dyspneic and diaphoretic and his systolic blood pressure decreased 34 mmHg. Because of these indicators of cardiac stress the work tolerance screening was discontinued. The client was asked to rest and his ECG, blood pressure and heart rate were monitored at two minute intervals. W. F.'s ECG and hemodynamics returned to levels within normal limits after ten minutes of rest. Subsequently another occupational therapy session was scheduled to review the results of the work tolerance screening with the client.

Recommendations

The following suggestions were made to W. F. to improve his performance on the job:

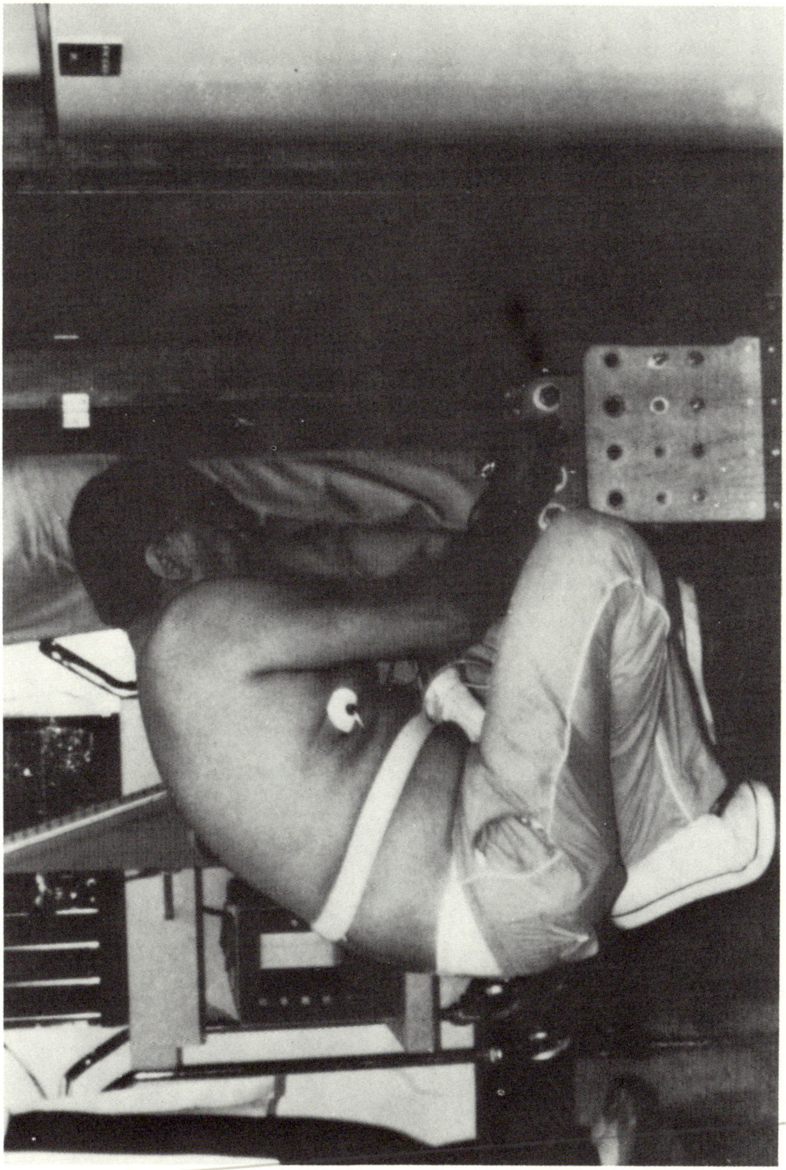

FIGURE 3.

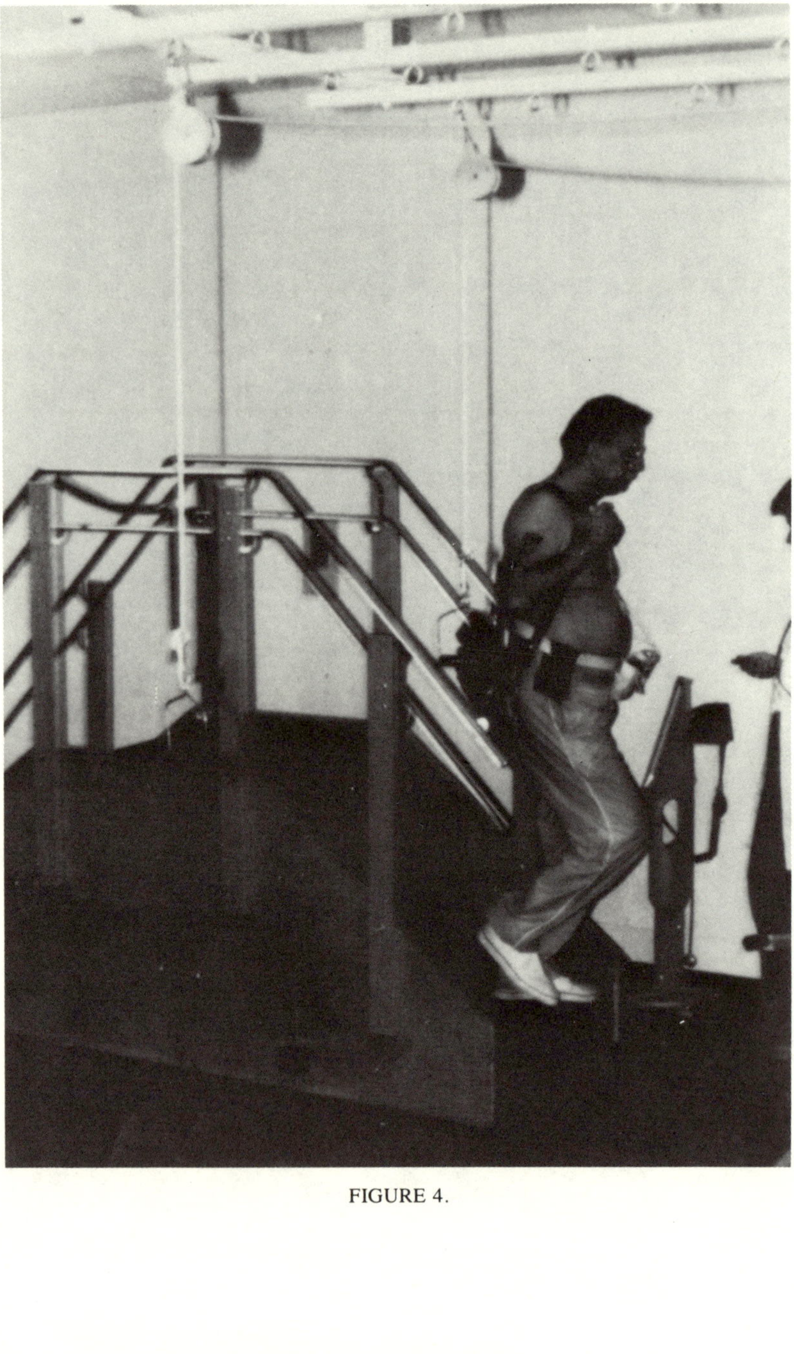

FIGURE 4.

1. Use another nearby elevator instead of stairs whenever possible.
2. Reduce speed of stair climbing to 30 steps per minute and rest between each flight of stairs.
3. Avoid becoming overly fatigued. Recovery from an activity should take less than one hour.
4. Try to reduce stress in the job by avoiding confrontation.
5. Be aware of symptoms of intolerance—sweating, shortness of breath, pain, fatigue.
6. Remember good body mechanics, i.e., bending at hips and knees, not waist.
7. Avoid extremes in temperature. In cold weather, wear a hat and muffler.

No special tools or equipment were suggested.

Results of the work tolerance screening were summarized and copies of the electrocardiogram and hemodynamic responses during and following the activity were sent to W. F.'s family physician.

Based on the physician's recommendations, the client returned to his job as an elevator repairman on a full-time basis.

SUMMARY

In a 3 week follow-up discussion with W. F. after his return to work, the client stated that he has incorporated many of the recommendations in his job, but states he continues to need to remind himself to "slow down" and to deal with the fact that he has had a heart attack. This he felt was particularly difficult being a supervisor who felt he must act as a model to younger employees.

The work tolerance screening has potential for further use as a supplement to the occupational therapy cardiac rehabilitation program. A proposal has been submitted for development of a Work Capacity Program in this setting.

REFERENCES

1. Hendrickson D, Anderson J, Gordon EE: A physiological approach to the regulation of activity in the cardiac convalescent. *Am J Occup Ther* 14: 292-296, 1960.

2. Ogden LD: Activity guidelines for early subacute and high-risk cardiac patients. *Am J Occup Ther* 33: 291-298, 1979.

3. Ogden LD: Hands on: Cardiac rehabilitation—guidelines for analysis and testing of activities of daily living with cardiac patients. *Physical Disabilities Specialty Section Newsletter* 3: 1-3, 1980.

4. Matheson LN, Ogden LD: *Work Tolerance Screening,* Trabuco Canyon, CA: Rehabilitation Institute of Southern California, 1983.

5. The MET is a measure of metabolic rate. One MET is equivalent to resting oxygen consumption.

6. U.S. Department of Labor: *Dictionary of Occupational Titles,* Washington, D.C.: U.S. Government Printing Office, 1977.

7. American College of Sports Medicine: *Guidelines for Graded Exercise Testing and Exercise Prescription,* Philadelphia, PA: Lea and Febiger, 1976.

8. Bennett GK: *Hand Tool Dexterity Test,* New York, NY: Psychological Corporation, 1965.

How to Improve Professional Reporting of Work Evaluations

Patricia Smith, MS, OTR
Julie S. Bohmfalk, MS, OTR

ABSTRACT. One of the significant hindrances to more frequent participation by occupational therapists in the vocational rehabilitation process is ineffective communication. The authors contend that occupational therapists conducting work evaluations can help overcome this deficit by making changes in the orientation, language, and form of their evaluation reports.

A recent research study by the authors comparing a survey of current occupational therapy practice and an assessment of needs of vocational rehabilitation counselors identified specific problems with work evaluation reports. These concerned uncertainty about who they were serving with their reports, use of language unfamiliar to persons not in the medical field, and presentation of data without interpretation or application to work situations.

The authors offer specific suggestions for writing reports of work evaluations which will provide better bases for helping workers return to their jobs.

Occupational therapists believe ability to work and feelings of self worth are closely linked since work is such a fundamental human function. This idea has been the basis of the profession's philosophy and has been reiterated at various times by prominent spokespersons in the profession.[1, 2] It has in the past led occupational therapists to involvement in prevocational evaluation and the vocational rehabilitation process. In recent years, however, as occupational therapists have tended to practice within the medical model work evaluation

---

Patricia Smith is Director of Occupational Assessment and Modification, Cupertino, California. Julie S. Bohmfalk is a hand therapist at Hand Therapy and Rehabilitation Associates, Inc., Los Gatos, California.

The authors gratefully acknowledge the assistance of Karen Diasio, MA, OTR, FAOTA, Professor, San Jose State University. They also extend appreciation to Thelma Wellerson Hook, MA, OTR, Director, Hand Therapy and Rehabilitation Associates, Inc., Los Gatos, California.

has become almost exclusively the function of a number of other professions. Now, however, there is a resurgence of interest among occupational therapists to be identified with the vocational rehabilitation process. This has led to the need to learn or to renew and sharpen some skills which are now becoming part of the educational preparation of other professionals.

Possibly the most significant hindrance to effective practice for occupational therapists in the vocational rehabilitation process is ineffective communication. A recent research study by the authors comparing an assessment of needs of vocational rehabilitation counselors and a survey of current occupational therapy practice in physical capacity assessment, revealed a number of opportunities to improve communication between therapists and their referral sources.[3] Some of these solutions are found in the effective use of the report of the evaluation.

PROBLEMS FOUND BY CLIENTS USING REPORTS FROM OCCUPATIONAL THERAPISTS

Occupational therapists' reports of work evaluations are often not as effective as they might be because therapists frequently fail to maintain an awareness of their accountability to the referring agent as the "customer". It is his needs that are to be met, not just the patient's needs. The evaluation report, therefore, is used most effectively when its content is aimed specifically to the customer/client and his needs. Although the therapist is evaluating a worker/patient, the client is the referring agent. That client is usually a vocational rehabilitation counselor, insurance carrier, rehabilitation coordinator, rehabilitation nurse, attorney, or others, none of whom are medical practitioners. In order to meet the specific needs of such clients the therapist must maintain an orientation to work and its demands throughout the evaluation process, and must report his findings in terms of work. Therapists used to communicating with other health care providers within a medical setting must now develop a skill for communicating with professionals with the orientation and vocabulary of work settings.

The research[3] revealed that because of extensive use of medical and kinesiologic terms by therapists, clients frequently do not understand the language or meaning of the occupational therapy reports. One experienced vocational counselor expressed to the authors the desire to see occupational therapists' reports in "baby talk". She remarked that she frequently has to ask occupational therapists for interpretation of their reports in language she can understand and relate to. Clients require reports written in clear language which conveys meaning without using medical and kinesiologic terms, occupational therapy jargon, or unfamiliar abbreviations. Reports that require interpretation do not serve the worker/patient or the profession well. Not only that, they create an inclination by users not to seek occupational therapy services and thereby avoid an additional expense for what might well be useless information.

It was found that reports contain few observations concerning work-related behavior and worker characteristics which occupational therapists are qualified to observe and evaluate. Clients expect reports of all significant clinical observations and opinions gathered during the evaluation process. Furthermore, the official position on work-related assessment of the American Occupational Therapy Association is that, in addition to evaluating "work abilities related to a specific job task", specific objectives of the prevocational evaluation include "assessing the client's learning abilities and retention of skills; evaluating . . . psychological and social factors such as . . . habits, and interpersonal qualities."[4, p 882] Though the therapist cannot be paid for time spent looking for data which was not specifically requested, ample opportunity should exist in most evaluation sessions to make observations of work-related behaviors and worker characteristics.

Often reports by occupational therapists of work-related evaluations consist of a number of pages of raw data which are not interpreted to show the ability of the worker/patient to perform work tasks. This tends to create the question of whether the information had been gathered by a technician, who reports only specific factual items, or by a professional who analyzes and interprets factual data and clinical observations.[5] Recipients of evaluation reports feel strongly that they are purchasing not simply factual information, but rather the therapist's analysis and interpretation and professional opinion regarding the worker's ability to function on the job.

REPORT MODIFICATIONS OF EVALUATION METHODS

Therapists may need to modify their assessment tools or procedures because of special needs or disabilities of the patient. One of the strengths occupational therapists have shown over the years has been the ability to arrange for and test persons who because of unusual or severe disability cannot be evaluated by standardized methods. Therapists thus may modify parts of their work evaluation procedures in order to gain an accurate picture of the capabilities of the worker being tested, or in order to answer specific questions from the referral source. Such modifications should be reported. By reporting instances when therapists do modify their assessment tools or procedures the therapist gives a more valid picture of the evaluation process. The report then also conveys by inference the unique contribution occupational therapists bring to the evaluative situation.[6]

As another important ingredient of the report the therapist should evaluate the need for and make recommendations for devices and work modifications that make job performance possible. Though not specifically requested, problem-solving suggestions to clients and/or employers should be thought of as a responsibility and special contribution of the occupational therapist. Also, if special devices are to be constructed the therapist can and should provide suggestions for cost-effective solutions, drawing on his experience with adaptive equipment and daily life functions. Funds for purchase or fabrication are frequently available, but may not be used because the "what to" and the "how to" are not known. Such situations can usually be solved by the occupational therapist.

FORM OF THE REPORT

In the American Journal of Occupational Therapy, Overs[7] gave some excellent suggestions for writing reports of work evaluations. He urged using a language structure for the report that combined two elements: specific factual items about performance and generalizations or deductions as to what they mean in work terms. Facts such as percentile ranks, range of motion measures, or indications of muscle weakness, can ordinarily be used as a part of a sentence in which a generalization is made about their effects. The facts are thus presented in such a way that their usefulness and applicability are apparent by relating the worker's condition to his work potential. The following statement provides an example of the two elements in combination. "Although Mr. Worker lacks 60 degrees of flexion in the left wrist, he is able to compensate for the loss when using tools by raising his elbow out to the side. He is able to work in confined spaces as long as he has approximately one foot of space to his left side." Use of the two elements in the suggested manner allows the evaluator to submit short reports with concise narrative format rather than with many worksheets. If requested scoresheets with specific data can be provided later. Nothing speaks louder and better than clear brief reports that respond to the client's needs.

RECOMMENDATIONS

The research and experience of the authors leads to the conclusion that occupational therapists could enhance the effectiveness of their reports of work evaluations in the following ways:

1. Maintain an awareness of who the customer/client is and what his needs are. Tailor your evaluation and report to that orientation.
2. Modify the evaluation process when necessary to gain an accurate picture of the worker's skills.
3. Tell the client when information has been gathered through non-standardized methods; otherwise, he will assume the worker can perform without modifications.
4. Recommend devices, adaptations, and modifications when you have found they would assist the injured worker to function on a job.
5. Remember that as a professional you as an occupational therapist are expected to report supportable opinion and observation.
6. Present integrated factual items and observations in concise narrative format rather than a collection of forms, checklists, and scoresheets. Examples and exact application to the worker make the content clearer.
7. Use easily understood, jargon-free language.

SUMMARY

In any evaluative situation the activity of collecting information has merit only "when the information is used to improve the planning and subsequent delivery of services."[8, p 2] Reports of work evaluations improve the planning and delivery of vocational rehabilitation services when they provide bases for problem-solving courses of action. To provide these bases they must be aimed at the clients' needs, written in easily understood language, and be related to the worker's ability to perform on the job. Your well-written reports will make a significant contribution toward returning workers to jobs.

REFERENCES

1. Cromwell FS: A procedure for pre-vocational evaluation. *Am J Occup Ther* 13: 1-4, 1959.

2. Wegg LS: Role of the occupational therapist in vocational rehabilitation. *Am J Occup Ther* 11: 252-254, 1957.

3. Smith P, Bohmfalk J: *Recommendations for improved occupational therapy practice in physical capacity assessment of the spinal cord injured person.* Unpublished Master's Thesis, San Jose State University, 1982.

4. Ellsworth P, Davy J, Mitcham M, Parkin J and Presseler S: The association-the role of occupational therapy in the vocational evaluation process. *Am J Occup Ther* 34: 881-883, 1980.

5. *Vocational evaluation project final report,* Vocational Evaluation and Work Adjustment Association, Menomonie, Wisconsin: Materials Development Center, 1975.

6. Esser TJ: *Effective report writing in vocational evaluation and work adjustment programs,* Menomonie, Wisconsin: Materials Development Center, 1974.

7. Overs R: Writing work evaluation reports: chore or challenge? *Am J Occup Ther* 18: 63-65, 1964.

8. Esser TJ: *Gathering information for evaluation planning,* Menomonie, Wisconsin: Materials Development Center, 1980.